SpringerBriefs in Modern Perspectives on Disability Research

This book series on disability research is a comprehensive collection of research on disability and related issues. The series is designed to promote interdisciplinary collaboration and exchange, bringing together scholars and practitioners from different fields to share their perspectives and insights. Disability research is an interdisciplinary field that examines the social, cultural, historical, and political dimensions of disability. It encompasses a wide range of topics, including disability rights, accessibility, assistive technologies, healthcare, education, employment, and social welfare. Disability research scholars employ a range of theoretical and methodological approaches to understand the experiences of people with disabilities, as well as the ways in which disability intersects with other social identities such as race, gender, sexuality, and class.

The series seeks to advance knowledge and understanding of disability by publishing rigorous, innovative, and relevant research. It aims to promote disability rights and social justice by highlighting the ways in which people with disabilities are marginalized and discriminated against in society, and advocating for greater social inclusion and accessibility. The series also seeks to inform policy and practice by disseminating research findings that can help to shape policy decisions and contribute to positive social change.

Gabriel Bennett

Understanding Hearing Loss

Exploring Perspectives and Strategies

Springer

Gabriel Bennett
c/o Dr. Matthew Bennett
Adelaide, SA, Australia

ISSN 3004-9709 ISSN 3004-9717 (electronic)
SpringerBriefs in Modern Perspectives on Disability Research
ISBN 978-981-95-1095-5 ISBN 978-981-95-1096-2 (eBook)
https://doi.org/10.1007/978-981-95-1096-2

This Springer imprint is published by the registered company Springer Nature Singapore Pte Ltd.
The registered company address is: 152 Beach Road, #21-01/04 Gateway East, Singapore 189721, Singapore

Preface

This book offers a comprehensive, evidence-based exploration of how hearing impairment affects individuals from early childhood through to late adulthood. Drawing on systematic reviews and meta-analyses, this volume examines clinical, communicative, cognitive, and social outcomes, as well as the diagnostic and environmental factors that shape experiences of hearing loss. With a particular focus on underserved and under-researched populations, it highlights critical gaps in our current knowledge while identifying opportunities for more inclusive, rigorous, and impactful research. This book is essential reading for researchers, clinicians, and policy-makers seeking to improve hearing health outcomes across diverse communities and life stages.

Adelaide, Australia

Gabriel Bennett

Competing Interests The author has no competing interests to declare that are relevant to the content of this manuscript.

Statement About the Use of Artificial Intelligence

ChatGPT, a large language model artificial intelligence program developed by the company OpenAI, was used to enhance the clarity of the concepts articulated in this book. All other procedures that were used to create this book were performed by Dr Gabriel Bennett.

Contents

About the Author

Gabriel Bennett, formally Dr Matthew Bennett, holds a PhD in Disability Studies from Flinders University, South Australia, Australia. He has lectured in Disability Studies at Griffith University, Queensland, Australia. He has also advised the Australian Government's Autism CRC and has published multiple books, including:

- Bennett, G., & Goodall, E. (2024). *The Role That Assistance Dogs Play in Supporting People with Disabilities*. Springer International Publishing AG. https://doi.org/10.1007/978-981-97-1492-6
- Bennett, G. (2024). *Senotherapy: A Potential Pharmacological Strategy for Prolonging Human Lifespan and Healthspan*. Springer International Publishing AG. https://doi.org/10.1007/978-981-97-3637-9
- Bennett, G. (2024). *A Scoping Review of Clinical Studies About the Therapeutic Benefits of Medical Cannabis*. Springer International Publishing AG. https://link.springer.com/book/9789819779406
- Bennett, G., & Goodall, E. (2024). *Autistic People With Co-occurring Psychological Conditions: Prevalence and Perspectives From Autistics, Their Families, and Professionals*. Springer International Publishing AG. https://doi.org/10.1007/978-981-97-0656-3

Abbreviations

ABR	Auditory brainstem response
AOHL	Adult-onset hearing loss
ARHL	Age-related hearing loss
CDC	Centers for Disease Control and Prevention
EcochG	Electrocochleography
HHL	Hidden hearing loss
HTLs	Hearing threshold levels
LEP	Limited English proficiency
MCI	Mild cognitive impairment
MEMR	Middle ear muscle reflex
NIHL	Noise-induced hearing loss
OME	Otitis media with effusion
PRISMA	Preferred Reporting Items for Systematic Reviews and Meta-Analyses
RCTs	Randomised controlled trials
STT	Speech-to-text
WHO	World Health Organization

Chapter 1
Introduction

1.1 Overview of Hearing Impairment

Hearing impairment, also known as hearing loss, refers to a partial or complete inability to perceive sounds in one or both ears. This condition can be present at birth (congenital) or develop later in life (acquired), and its severity can range from mild difficulties in hearing soft sounds to profound deafness, where even very loud noises may not be detected (Centers for Disease Control and Prevention [CDC], 2024; World Health Organization [WHO], 2024). The impact of hearing impairment depends not only on its degree but also on the age of onset, whether one or both ears are affected, and whether the loss is stable, progressive, or fluctuating (CDC, 2024).

There are several types of hearing loss, each with distinct causes and characteristics. Conductive hearing loss occurs when sound waves are prevented from reaching the inner ear due to problems in the outer or middle ear, such as ear infections, fluid buildup, or structural abnormalities. This type of loss is sometimes reversible through medical or surgical intervention (CDC, 2024; Johns Hopkins Medicine, 2024). Sensorineural hearing loss, the most common type, results from damage to the inner ear (cochlea) or the auditory nerve. It is typically permanent and can be caused by ageing, prolonged noise exposure, certain medications, or illnesses (Healthy Hearing, 2025). Mixed hearing loss is a combination of both conductive and sensorineural components, while auditory neuropathy spectrum disorder involves a disruption in the way the inner ear or auditory nerve transmits sound signals to the brain (CDC, 2024).

The degree of hearing loss is also important in understanding its impact. Mild hearing loss may make it difficult to hear soft or distant sounds, while moderate loss can interfere with understanding normal speech, especially in noisy environments. Severe hearing loss means only very loud sounds are audible, and profound loss or deafness may result in no sound perception at all (WHO, 2024). Additional

G. Bennett, *Understanding Hearing Loss*, SpringerBriefs in Modern Perspectives on Disability Research,
https://doi.org/10.1007/978-981-95-1096-2_1

descriptors include whether the loss is unilateral (one ear) or bilateral (both ears), symmetrical or asymmetrical, and whether it occurs before (pre-lingual) or after (post-lingual) language development (CDC, 2024).

Hearing impairment is a widespread condition, affecting over 1.5 billion people worldwide, with around 430 million experiencing disabling hearing loss (WHO, 2024). The prevalence increases with age; approximately 30% of adults older than 60 years of age are affected. Congenital hearing loss is estimated to occur in 1 to 3 per 1000 live births in developed countries and as many as 6 per 1000 in developing nations (CDC, 2023). By 2050, it is projected that over 700 million people will require some form of hearing rehabilitation (WHO, 2024).

Living with hearing impairment can present daily challenges. Individuals may struggle to communicate, particularly in noisy environments or group settings, which can lead to frustration and social withdrawal (Marschark & Hauser, 2021). Children with hearing loss often experience delayed language development, which can impact their academic performance and social integration (Yoshinaga-Itano, 2003). Adults may face barriers to employment, education, and accessing public services if appropriate accommodations are not available (WHO, 2024). The psychological effects can be significant, with an increased risk of isolation, depression, and reduced self-esteem, especially among older adults (Mener et al., 2013).

Despite these challenges, a variety of supports and solutions can greatly improve quality of life for those with hearing impairments. Early detection through newborn screening and routine hearing tests is vital, as timely intervention can support language and cognitive development (CDC, 2023). Technological advancements such as hearing aids, cochlear implants, and bone-anchored hearing devices have transformed the management of hearing loss, enabling many people to participate more fully in daily life (WHO, 2024). Communication supports, including sign language, speech therapy, aural rehabilitation, and captioning services, help bridge communication gaps (Marschark & Hauser, 2021). Environmental modifications—like reducing background noise, using visual alarms, and providing written or visual information—can make public spaces more accessible (Yoshinaga-Itano, 2003). Education, advocacy, and public awareness campaigns are also essential for promoting inclusion and reducing stigma (WHO, 2024). Importantly, up to half of all hearing loss cases are preventable through public health measures such as immunisation, safe listening practices, and avoiding exposure to ototoxic medications (WHO, 2024).

In summary, hearing impairment is a complex and prevalent condition with far-reaching effects on communication, education, and social participation. Understanding the different types and degrees of hearing loss, along with the daily challenges faced by those affected, underscores the importance of early intervention, technological solutions, supportive environments, and prevention strategies in improving outcomes and quality of life.

1.2 Research Questions

To investigate the literature about the impact of hearing loss the following research questions are explored in this book:

- Question 1—*"How effective are current clinical, technological, and communicative interventions in addressing the needs and outcomes of people with hearing loss across different life stages?"*
- Question 2—*"What are the diagnostic approaches and risk factors associated with hearing loss across diverse populations and environments?"*
- Question 3—*"What is the impact of hearing loss across the lifespan on cognitive, psychological, developmental, and health outcomes?"*

1.3 Search Procedures for Relevant Citations

On 19 May 2025 a keyword search of the term *"hearing impairment"* in the article's title for articles on PubMed was conducted. All articles were restricted to English and had to have been published between 1 January 2020 and 19 May 2025. This search approach yielded more than 6500 unique citations, which was beyond the ability of the researcher to examine each citation. To mitigate this problem only systematic literature reviews and meta-analyses were filtered from the results (see Appendix A). This search strategy was used, in part, because it was assumed that the authors of such studies would have collated studies that were not indexed on PubMed.

1.4 Methodological Strengths and Weaknesses of This Study

1.4.1 Methodological Strengths

High-quality evidence: Systematic reviews and meta-analyses are sometimes regarded as the most robust forms of evidence within the hierarchy of research, especially in disciplines like health, psychology, and education. Systematic literature reviews apply rigorous, transparent methodologies for identifying, selecting, and appraising primary studies, ensuring that their conclusions are based on comprehensive and unbiased data. Meta-analyses go a step further by statistically pooling results from multiple studies, which enhances the power and precision of findings. By relying on these high-quality sources, the results in this book come from some of the most credible and validated evidence available.

Comprehensive aggregation of research: Systematic literature reviews and meta-analyses aggregate a wide range of primary research, often encompassing dozens or even hundreds of individual studies. They consolidate findings into overarching patterns, clarify areas of consensus and disagreement, and sometimes explore changes across time or population groups. This means that instead of evaluating each primary study individually, this book has drawn from expertly curated synthesis that already reflects a broad spectrum of research. As a result, this book offers an efficient yet expansive overview of the field, covering far more ground than would be feasible using only primary literature.

Methodologically robust research: Systematic literature reviews and meta-analyses are typically guided by predefined protocols, including structured search strategies, explicit inclusion and exclusion criteria, and critical quality assessments of included studies. These procedures reduce the likelihood of selection bias and enhance transparency making the results more reliable and reproducible. This methodological clarity adds to the overall trustworthiness of this book's conclusions, reinforcing its value for readers seeking knowledge about evidence-based insights.

Identification of research gaps and inconsistencies: A key feature of systematic literature reviews is their capacity to identify limitations within the existing literature. They often conclude with an analysis of research gaps, methodological weaknesses, or under-represented populations. This makes such studies especially useful for highlighting where further investigation is needed and where inconsistencies persist. This book has used these insights to map the current boundaries of knowledge in hearing impairment research and propose directions of inquiry in the future.

Relevance across disciplines: Systematic literature reviews and meta-analyses are not confined to clinical disciplines—they appear in fields ranging from public health and education to disability studies, linguistics, and social policy. This interdisciplinary applicability allows readers the opportunity to draw on a wide-ranging body of literature without sacrificing any methodological rigour. By integrating findings from diverse domains, this book can offer a truly comprehensive perspective that appeals to varied audiences while maintaining scholarly coherence.

Time efficiency and manageability: Given the vast scope of hearing impairment research, attempting to review all primary studies would have been both impractical and overwhelming. Focusing exclusively on systematic literature reviews and meta-analyses significantly streamlines this process. The authors of the systematic literature reviews and meta-analyses have already filtered and evaluated primary research, making it possible for the reader to develop a coherent synthesis without becoming bogged down by the sheer volume and variability of individual studies.

1.4.2 Methodological Weaknesses

Risk of omitting emerging or niche topics: Systematic literature reviews and meta-analyses take time to conduct and publish, so they often lag current research trends. As a result, emerging findings, cutting-edge interventions, or new theoretical perspectives may not yet be captured in existing reviews. Similarly, niche or under-researched topics—such as minority language users with hearing impairments or intersectional analyses—might not be synthesised at all, leading to gaps.

Loss of primary data: While meta-analyses provide powerful generalisations, they often simplify the complexity of individual studies. Important contextual details—such as participant experiences, variations in study design, or qualitative findings—can be lost or excluded in pursuit of aggregated results. This may result in a lack of detail, including lived experiences, social dynamics, or culturally specific issues related to hearing impairments.

Potential over-representation of clinical and quantitative paradigms: Systematic literature reviews and meta-analyses are more common in clinical and quantitative research, where standardised outcomes allow for statistical synthesis. As a result, these methodologies often overrepresent biomedical, treatment-based, or impairment-focused perspectives. More interpretive, community-based, or qualitative research—especially common in disability studies and deaf culture—may be under-represented or entirely excluded. This can result in a bias towards medicalised narratives and marginalised sociocultural viewpoints.

1.5 Intended Audience for This Book

Clinicians and allied health professionals: This book can be of value to audiologists, speech-language pathologists, general practitioners, and allied health professionals who support individuals diagnosed with hearing impairments. By summarising a broad range of literature—from audiological science and medical interventions to the psychological and social consequences of hearing loss—it provides these professionals with a comprehensive, evidence-informed foundation for understanding hearing loss. This book also has the potential to support clinical decision-making and holistic care planning by contextualising hearing impairment not only as a medical condition but also as a lived experience that is influenced by communications, culture, and community.

Researchers and academics: For scholars and academic researchers from various disciplines—including audiology, psychology, disability studies, education, and neuroscience—this book provides a valuable synthesis of the existing body of knowledge about hearing impairments. This book identifies key debates, emerging trends, and research gaps, enabling readers the opportunity to position their studies within broader scholarly conventions. Whether used as a foundational resource in teaching, a springboard for new investigations, or a citation-rich companion for writing, this book contributes to advancing multidisciplinary dialogue around hearing and deafness.

Health policy-makers and public health officials: Policy-makers and public health professionals will find this book a useful resource for understanding the economic and societal implications of hearing impairments. By drawing from both clinical and sociocultural literature, this book provides a nuanced overview of the barriers to care, disparities in outcomes, and cost-effectiveness of early intervention strategies. This book can help inform the development of inclusive health policies, national hearing strategies, and equity-focused funding models, ensuring that interventions are not only evidence-based but socially and culturally responsive.

People with hearing impairments and their families: This book can serve people who are deaf or who experience difficulties with hearing, as well as their families and carers, by offering a clear summary of the research that affects their lives. Through simple and accessible language, along with thoughtful framing, it illuminates the various ways hearing loss is understood, experienced, and addressed—medically, socially, and politically. Readers will find not only information about treatment options and assistive technology, but also representation and validation of their lived experiences.

Technology developers: Engineers and product developers working on hearing-related technologies—such as hearing aids, cochlear implants, real-time captioning, or auditory training apps—will find this book a valuable user-centred resource. By mapping the intersections between clinical evidence, user experience, and emerging technologies, this book helps developers better understand the functional needs and diverse preferences of people with hearing impairments. This book supports innovation that is not only technologically sound but grounded in the lived realities of end-users.

Advocacy groups and disability organisations: For advocacy organisations and disability support services, this book provides a rich source of empirical evidence and conceptual frameworks to guide their work. Whether used in community education, policy advocacy, or program development, the insights offered will strengthen their capacity to advocate effectively for the rights and inclusion of people with hearing impairments. By articulating the connections between hearing loss, social participation, legal recognition, and accessibility, this book affirms the centrality of hearing issues in broader disability discourse.

Mental health professionals and counsellors: Hearing impairment is often linked to increased rates of depression, social isolation, and cognitive decline. Psychologists, counsellors, and social workers can use this book to better understand the psychological and emotional impacts of hearing loss and to develop more empathic, tailored approaches to therapy and support. The insights in this book can also inform training modules for mental health professionals working in rehabilitation or geriatric settings.

Aged care providers and gerontologists: Age-related hearing loss is highly prevalent, and its management is crucial for quality of life among older populations. Aged care providers, nursing home staff, and researchers in gerontology would benefit from the synthesis of literature on hearing impairments in older adults that is presented in this book, particularly where it intersects with dementia, cognitive decline, and communication challenges in care settings.

1.6 Description of Upcoming Chapters

1.6.1 Chapter 2: Needs and Outcomes of People with Hearing Loss Across Different Life Stages

Hearing loss is a significant public health issue affecting individuals across all life stages, with clinical, social, and communicative implications. Despite increasing recognition of its impact, disparities persist in diagnosis, management, and support—particularly in healthcare and education. This chapter explores how effectively current interventions—clinical, technological, and communicative—meet the needs of people with hearing loss. It synthesises findings from six systematic reviews covering early childhood to late adulthood, focusing on linguistic interventions, assistive technologies, communication strategies, and service uptake. Special attention is given to under-researched groups, including those with subclinical hearing loss and limited English proficiency. Key themes include communication, accessibility, and intervention efficacy.

1.6.2 Chapter 3: Diagnostic Approaches and Risk Factors Associated with Hearing Loss Across Diverse Populations and Environments

Hearing loss is a complex global health issue that is influenced by environmental, occupational, and sociodemographic factors. Recent reviews highlight diagnostic challenges and risk factors across diverse settings—rural farms, industrial sites, gaming environments, and clinical contexts. In this chapter, special attention is given to under-recognised groups such as farmworkers, children with sensorineural hearing loss, and gamers, as well as conditions like hidden hearing loss and balance disorders. The findings underscore the need for improved diagnostics, inclusive research, and scalable interventions for at-risk populations.

1.6.3 Chapter 4: Hearing Loss Across the Lifespan and Cognitive, Psychological, Developmental, and Health Outcomes

Hearing loss affects individuals across all stages of life and carries implications that extend far beyond sensory impairment. Recent research has increasingly focused on the cognitive, psychological, and psychosocial consequences of hearing loss, highlighting its role as a significant public health concern. Across childhood, adulthood, and older age, hearing impairment has been linked to a range of adverse outcomes, including developmental delays, academic challenges, social isolation, depression, and increased risk of cognitive decline and dementia. Systematic reviews and meta-analyses conducted across diverse populations and global regions have begun to illuminate these complex relationships. Notably, studies have revealed that early intervention, communicative competence, and hearing aid use are critical protective factors, while comorbidities such as cardiovascular disease, depression, and social disadvantage may amplify risk. Despite these insights, gaps in research persist—particularly concerning under-represented populations and the need for longitudinal, biomarker-informed investigations. Together, these findings underscore the urgent need for integrated, lifespan-oriented approaches to hearing care that account for cognitive, emotional, and social well-being. Early identification and tailored interventions can not only improve communication but also serve as a foundation for mitigating long-term developmental and neurodegenerative risks. Moving forward, more representative and methodologically rigorous studies are required to strengthen the evidence base and inform policy, education, and clinical practice in hearing health and beyond.

1.6.4 Chapter 5: Opportunities for Research in the Future

Over the past several decades, research on hearing loss has grown substantially, offering important knowledge about its prevalence, underlying causes, and wide-ranging psychosocial effects. Yet, the reliability and generalisability of this research are often limited by recurring methodological challenges found across systematic reviews, meta-analyses, and original studies. This chapter highlights the most frequently observed limitations in the existing literature, such as study design weaknesses, various forms of bias, inconsistent measurement approaches, and analytical shortcomings. By critically exploring these issues, this chapter aims to equip researchers, clinicians, and policy-makers with a deeper understanding of the evidence base's current limitations and to guide more rigorous, impactful research in the future.

1.6.5 Chapter 6: Closing Remarks

This concluding chapter emphasises the broad and complex impact of hearing loss across all life stages, highlighting significant gaps in current diagnosis, intervention, and research. It underscores the need for inclusive, culturally sensitive, and lifespan-oriented approaches to hearing care that address not only clinical symptoms but also social and psychological outcomes. This chapter calls attention to methodological limitations in existing research that hinder progress and stresses the importance of rigorous, representative studies going forward. Ultimately, it advocates for collaborative efforts among researchers, clinicians, policy-makers, and communities to develop equitable, effective strategies that improve the lives of people with hearing loss worldwide.

References

Centers for Disease Control and Prevention. (2023). *Hearing loss in children*. https://www.cdc.gov/ncbddd/hearingloss/data.html

Centers for Disease Control and Prevention. (2024). *Types of hearing loss*. https://www.cdc.gov/ncbddd/hearingloss/types.html

Healthy Hearing. (2025). *Types and degrees of hearing loss*. https://www.healthyhearing.com/help/hearing-loss/types

Johns Hopkins Medicine. (2024). *Conductive hearing loss*. https://www.hopkinsmedicine.org/health/conditions-and-diseases/conductive-hearing-loss

Marschark, M., & Hauser, P. C. (2021). *Deaf cognition: Foundations and outcomes*. Oxford University Press.

Mener, D. J., Betz, J., Genther, D. J., Chen, D., & Lin, F. R. (2013). Hearing loss and depression in older adults. *Journal of the American Geriatrics Society, 61*(9), 1627–1629. https://doi.org/10.1111/jgs.12429

World Health Organization. (2024). *Deafness and hearing loss*. https://www.who.int/news-room/fact-sheets/detail/deafness-and-hearing-loss

Yoshinaga-Itano, C. (2003). Early intervention after universal neonatal hearing screening: Impact on outcomes. *Mental Retardation and Developmental Disabilities Research Reviews, 9*(4), 252–266. https://doi.org/10.1002/mrdd.10088

Chapter 2
Needs and Outcomes of People with Hearing Loss Across Different Life Stages

2.1 Needs of People with Hearing Impairments/Hearing Loss

Vocabulary, grammar, and discourse represent discrete yet interdependent components of linguistic competence in early adulthood. Current research consistently demonstrates that children diagnosed with hearing loss often exhibit delays or deficits in language development when compared to their hearing peers. Arráez Vera et al. (2025) published a systematic literature review and two meta-analyses in which they critically assessed the efficacy of targeted linguistic interventions aimed at enhancing oral discourse abilities among children who were hearing impaired. They conducted their systematic literature review in accordance with the Preferred Reporting Items for Systematic Reviews and Meta-Analyses (PRISMA) 2020 guidelines, encompassing five major academic databases. In total, 23 studies met their inclusion criteria and were subsequently incorporated into the qualitative synthesis. Of these collected studies, 12 contained sufficient quantitative data to be included in their successive meta-analyses. Two distinct meta-analyses were conducted: addressing the macrostructural and microstructural dimensions of oral discourse, respectively. Findings from this review support the efficacy of linguistic interventions in promoting oral discourse development among children with hearing loss. Notably, many of these interventions incorporate visual aids and explicit grammatical instruction. However, given the relatively small number of studies included and the high degree of heterogeneity measured, the generalisability of these findings remains limited. Further research into employing rigorous, standardised methodologies is warranted to strengthen the evidence base.

People who present both LEP and hearing loss encounter significant communication barriers, which are not always adequately addressed by conventional interpreter services. Although no established consensus exists regarding the most effective communication resources for this population. Speech-to-text (STT) applications incorporating translation functionalities may offer a promising alternative.

G. Bennett, *Understanding Hearing Loss*, SpringerBriefs in Modern Perspectives on Disability Research,
https://doi.org/10.1007/978-981-95-1096-2_2

To address this query, Ferraro et al. (2024) examined the current literature on the clinical applications of STT translation technologies and commercially available STT tools. They conducted a systematic literature review of English-language, peer-reviewed studies investigating the use of STT translation technologies in clinical contexts. In parallel, a comprehensive search was performed to identify STT software platforms commercially available. They reviewed studies that were published on PubMed, Medline, Embase, and Web of Science. Of the 591 unique citations that they screened, seven met the criteria for inclusion in their review. Additionally, 29 distinct STT translation applications were identified supporting translation across up to 140 languages. Stakeholder feedback reflected generally favourable perceptions of these tools. Key facilitators of implementation included their feasibility in terms of time and cost, while primary barriers encompassed risks of mistranslation and the difficulty of verifying translational accuracy. While ongoing advances in machine learning continue to enhance the development of STT technologies, there remains a notable gap in the literature specifically addressing their applicability for people with hearing loss.

Ferraro et al. concluded that preliminary evidence from small-scale studies indicates that STT translation applications may achieve an acceptable degree of accuracy when employed as adjuncts to standard clinical communication practices Further research should seek to address current implementation challenges, with particular emphasis on the dual needs of patients with both LEP and hearing loss. Furthermore, continued technological innovation and targeted evaluation are essential for optimising the use of STT translation tools.

Subclinical hearing loss, often defined as hearing impairment that does not meet the clinical thresholds for diagnosis yet results in perceptible communication difficulties, represents an under-recognised and frequently under-treated condition. People with subclinical hearing loss may experience reduced speech perception, especially in noisy environments, and encounter challenges in everyday listening situations, despite having audiometric thresholds within the "*normal*" range. Unlike those with clinically defined hearing loss, this population often falls outside the scope of traditional audiological intervention pathways, leading to low rates of help-seeking and minimal engagement with hearing health services. In this context, understanding behavioural responses to hearing difficulties—such as help-seeking—and evaluating the effectiveness of early intervention strategies, including the use of hearing devices, is of growing clinical importance. Frisby et al. (2024) published a systematic literature review that attempted to evaluate the current evidence on help-seeking behaviour, hearing device uptake, and hearing health outcomes, among people with subclinical hearing loss.

Frisby et al. conducted a structured search of three electronic databases—CINAHL, Medline (PubMed), and Scopus—in which they identified nine studies that met their inclusion criteria. The methodological quality of the studies was assessed using the National Institutes of Health Quality Assessment Tool, and the level of evidence was determined based on the centre for Evidence-Based Medicine classification framework. All studies included in their systematic literature review focused on adult participants. Three studies addressed help-seeking behaviour, identifying key determinants such as self-reported hearing difficulty, reduced speech-in-noise performance, and emotional responses to hearing-related challenges. Six studies evaluated the use of hearing devices, including conventional hearing aids ($n = 4$), hearables ($n = 1$), and frequency modulation systems ($n = 1$). These interventions were associated with improvements in perceived hearing ability, enhanced speech-in-noise understanding, and increased motivation to address hearing problems. However, none of the included studies explicitly examined the rate of hearing device uptake or factors influencing adoption. The overall methodological quality of the studies was limited, with variability in study design and levels of evidence.

Preliminary findings from Frisby et al.'s systematic literature review suggest that hearing devices may provide meaningful benefits for people with subclinical hearing loss, particularly in improving self-perceived auditory functioning and communication outcomes. Nonetheless, the evidence base remains limited by methodological weaknesses and an absence of focused research on device uptake and longitudinal outcomes. Investigations in the future should prioritise well-designed studies that explore help-seeking pathways, diagnostic practices, treatment decision-making, and the sustained effectiveness of interventions within this under-explored population.

Age-related hearing loss (ARHL) is one of the most prevalent chronic conditions affecting older adults globally, with significant implications for communication, social participation, cognitive function, and overall quality of life. Despite the availability of effectively auditory technologies such as hearing aids, challenges persist in achieving optimal rehabilitation outcomes due to a range of technological, clinical, and individual-level factors. The objective of Morvan et al.'s (2024) systematic review was to identify and synthesise the key factors contributing to the effective management of ARHL through hearing rehabilitation strategies.

Morvan et al.'s systematic review was conducted in accordance with the PRISMA 2020 guidelines. During May 2024 systematic searches were performed in four major electronic databases—Scopus, PubMed, Web of Science, and the Cochrane Library. Only peer-reviewed articles published between January 2005 and May 2024 were considered. Two independent reviewers assessed the retrieved studies for eligibility, and methodological quality was appraised using the Crowe Critical Appraisal Tool.

From an initial pool of 278 identified articles, 54 met the inclusion criteria and were included in their final analysis. Three overarching factors emerged as central to the effective use of hearing aids in the rehabilitation of ARHL:

1. *Signal processing technologies*: Advanced hearing aid features—such as directional microphones and noise reduction software—were found to significantly enhance user comfort and reduced speech intelligibility in noisy environments.
2. *Hearing aid fitting and prescription protocols*: Proper hearing aid fitting, particularly when guided by the National Acoustic Laboratories prescription rules, was shown to be essential for achieving optimal auditory outcomes. Bilateral

fittings and high-performing devices were associated with improved spatial localisation and noise discrimination capabilities.
3. *Patient-centred rehabilitation approaches*: Individualised patient-centred rehabilitation processes were identified as a critical success factor. This includes the use of patient-reported outcome measures, structured questionnaires, counselling interventions, and routine follow-up consultations. These strategies help address patient expectations, promote adherence, and improve satisfaction with rehabilitation outcomes.

While consensus regarding optimal acoustic parameters remains elusive—due in part to interindividual variability in audiological performance—the evidence underscores the importance of integrating both technological precision and patient-centred care in the rehabilitation of ARHL. Tailoring rehabilitation efforts to individual needs, fostering active patient participation, and employing structured outcome assessments are essential to improving hearing-related quality of life in this population. Research in the future should prioritise longitudinal, high-quality studies to refine fitting protocols and further validate patient engagement strategies.

Hearing loss represents a significant public health concern globally, with adverse effects on communication, social participation, mental health, and quality of life, in low- and middle-income countries, including Malaysia. Furthermore, the burden of untreated hearing loss is compounded by limitations in service accessibility, affordability, and public awareness. Despite the availability of diagnostic and rehabilitative hearing service, evidence suggests persistently low utilisation rates for hearing services in Malaysia. Romli et al. (2024) attempted to identify existing knowledge gaps concerning access to and outcomes from adult hearing care services in Malaysia. They searched for articles from four electronic databases—PubMed, CINAHL, Embase, and Scopus—resulting in 1261 records. An additional seven studies were identified through grey literature sources. Following the removal of duplicates, 647 records were screened by title and abstract. Based on the eligibility criteria, five studies were included in their final analysis.

Romli et al. reported that audiologists in Malaysia provided a broad spectrum of hearing care services, encompassing diagnostic assessments, hearing aid fittings, provision of assistive listening devices, auditory trainings, and counselling. Despite the range of services offered, the uptake of hearing healthcare services remained markedly low. Hearing aid usage rates were estimated at 2.7–4.4% among adults with at least mild hearing loss, and 6.5–7.3% among those with at least moderate hearing loss. Notably, none of the included studies provided outcome data regarding the effectiveness or impact of these hearing services.

Romli et al.'s research underscores a critical gap between the availability of hearing care services and their utilisation by adults in Malaysia. Their findings highlight a paucity of data regarding both the outcomes of hearing interventions and the underlying factors contributing to poor service uptake. Addressing the burden of hearing loss in Malaysia necessitates urgent and targeted efforts to:

1. Identify barriers to accessing care.
2. Enhance public and professional awareness.

3. Expand service delivery models.
4. Systematically evaluate the effectiveness of adult hearing care interventions within the Malaysian healthcare context.

Effective communication between healthcare professionals and patients is foundational to the delivery of safe, equitable, and high-quality healthcare. For people with hearing loss communication challenges can significantly impede access to appropriate care, understanding of medical information, adherence to treatment plans, and overall patient satisfaction. Despite increasing recognition of the importance of inclusive communication strategies, healthcare systems continue to underutilise available accommodations, such as assistive technologies and professional interpretation services. Weerapol and Leelakanok (2024) systematically reviewed published evidence regarding the communication methods used between healthcare professionals and patients with hearing loss. The objective of their research was to determine the prevalence of different communication modalities and assess the extent to which inclusive communication practices are implemented in healthcare settings. They searched for relevant studies across five major databases—Medline/PubMed, Scopus, CINHL, ScienceDirect, and Thai Journals Online complete. Eligible studies included those reporting on communication practices between healthcare professionals and adult patients with any degree of hearing loss. Data extraction focused on the prevalence and types of communication modes employed. A meta-analysis was performed using a random-effects model to account for heterogeneity among studies.

Weerapol and Leelakanok identified 20 studies that met the inclusion criteria for their systematic review. The most reported modes of communication were the use of hearing aids and gestures. The findings also highlighted a notable deficiency in healthcare professionals' capacity to communicate using sign language and limited access to qualified sign language interpreters across clinical environments. These authors concluded that substantial communication barriers persist for patients with hearing loss in healthcare settings. While hearing aids and non-verbal cues such as gestures are commonly used, these approaches are often inadequate to ensure effective, patient-centred communication. Their study also underscores the need to integrate qualified sign language interpreters and assistive communication technologies into routine clinical practice. Enhancing healthcare providers' training in inclusive communication and ensuring institutional support for accessible communication tools are essential steps towards improving health equity for patients with hearing impairments.

2.2 Conclusion

Taken together, these six reviews reveal both significant advancements and enduring limitations in how clinical, technological, and communicative interventions address the needs of people with hearing loss. Linguistic interventions targeting children have shown efficacy in improving oral discourse, particularly when visual and grammatical supports are integrated, although high heterogeneity among studies limits generalisability. Similarly, in older adults, successful auditory rehabilitation depends not only on advanced signal processing but also on personalised, patient-centred care that fosters adherence and satisfaction.

Emerging technologies, such as speech-to-text translation tools, offer promising solutions for populations with complex communicative needs, such as individuals with both LEP and hearing loss. However, questions about accuracy, user trust, and practical implementation remain. Subclinical hearing loss—frequently overlooked—presents another area of unmet need, with evidence suggesting that early device intervention may be beneficial, despite low help-seeking rates and limited longitudinal data. In Malaysia and comparable settings, structural barriers continue to impede access to adult hearing care, despite a diverse range of services being technically available.

A recurring theme across all studies is the persistent under-utilisation of inclusive communication strategies within healthcare, particularly the use of qualified sign language interpreters and assistive technologies. Even where tools and policies exist, the lack of provider training and systemic support undermines equitable care. Future research must prioritise methodologically rigorous studies, especially in under-represented populations and contexts. Furthermore, policy responses must be intersectional—addressing not only technological access but also language proficiency, cultural competence, and system-wide accountability.

In conclusion, while the existing evidence base affirms the potential of various interventions, it also underscores the urgent need for comprehensive, equitable, and inclusive strategies that respond to the complex realities of living with hearing loss across the lifespan.

References

Arráez Vera, G., Gonzálvez, C., & Ros, N. A. (2025). The effectiveness of linguistic intervention in children with hearing loss: A systematic review and meta-analysis. *Journal of Speech, Language, and Hearing Research, 68*(5), 2656–2673. https://doi.org/10.1044/2025_JSLHR-24-00589

Ferraro, T., Samaha, N. L., Tannan, U., Sookram, S., Wong, K., & Hwa, T. P. (2024). Use of speech-to-text translation resources to address communication barriers in patients with hearing loss: A systematic review. *Otology and Neurotology, 45*(9), 961–970. https://doi.org/10.1097/MAO.0000000000004272

Frisby, C., Oosthuizen, I., Manchaiah, V., & Swanepoel, W. (2024). Hearing help-seeking, hearing device uptake and hearing health outcomes in individuals with subclinical hearing loss: A systematic review. *International Journal of Audiology, 63*(12), 925–935. https://doi.org/10.1080/14992027.2024.2311660

Morvan, P., Buisson-Savin, J., Boiteux, C., Bailly-Masson, E., Buhl, M., & Thai-Van, H. (2024). Factors in the effective use of hearing aids among subjects with age-related hearing loss: A systematic review. *Journal of Clinical Medicine, 13*(14), 4027. https://doi.org/10.3390/jcm13144027

Romli, M., Timmer, B. H. B., & Dawes, P. (2024). Hearing care services for adults with hearing loss in Malaysia: A scoping review. *International Journal of Audiology, 63*(10), 753–760. https://doi.org/10.1080/14992027.2023.2270594

Weerapol, N., & Leelakanok, N. (2024). Communication between healthcare professionals and patients with hearing loss: A systematic review and meta-analysis. *American Journal of Health-system Pharmacy: AJHP: Official Journal of the American Society of Health-System Pharmacists, 81*(12), 521–530. https://doi.org/10.1093/ajhp/zxae045

Chapter 3
Diagnostic Approaches and Risk Factors Associated with Hearing Loss Across Diverse Populations and Environments

3.1 Diagnostic Approaches and Risk Factors Associated with Hearing Loss

An examination of the citations retrieved from PubMed revealed seven studies that were deemed to answer the research question *"What are the diagnostic approaches and risk factors associated with hearing loss across diverse populations and environments?"* (Coco et al., 2025; Dillrd et al., 2024; Firle & Richter, 2025; Kitoh et al., 2024; Makaruse et al., 2025; Shenoy et al., 2025; Xu et al., 2024). What follows now is a description of the contents of these studies, including their results. These studies are grouped into the following two thematic categories: risk factors associated with hearing loss and diagnostic approaches.

3.1.1 Risk Factors Associated with Hearing Loss

Noise-induced hearing loss (NIHL) remains one of the most prevalent occupational health issues globally. In Germany, it is recognised as the most reported occupational disease. While NIHL is frequently associated with industrial settings, professional musicians—particularly those performing classical music—are also exposed to potentially harmful sound levels during rehearsals and performances. Despite growing awareness, the true prevalence and characteristics of hearing loss among musicians remain unclear due to the diversity of study designs and populations. To address this gap, Firle and Richter (2025) undertook a scoping review to assess the prevalence, audiometric characteristics, and genre-specific patterns of hearing loss among professional musicians. They examined articles published on MEDLINE,

G. Bennett, *Understanding Hearing Loss*, SpringerBriefs in Modern Perspectives on Disability Research,
https://doi.org/10.1007/978-981-95-1096-2_3

Embase, the Cochrane Library, and Google Scholar. Only original studies reporting audiometric testing results were included in their analysis.

Seventy-nine studies met Firle and Richter's inclusion criteria and were included in their descriptive synthesis. The median sample size was 52 participants, with most studies comprising people with a minimum of five years' experience as active musicians. Many studies focused on students, resulting in a notable paucity of data about older or retired musicians and precluding reliable estimates of lifetime prevalence. Audiometric data revealed an elevated risk of hearing loss exceeding 15–20 decibel (dB) in the 4000–6000 hertz (Hz) range among classical musicians, although normal hearing was also reported in this cohort. Rock, pop, and jazz musicians exhibited a heightened risk of hearing loss exceeding 20 dB within the broader frequency range of 3000–8000 Hz. Evidence for other genres, such as military, marching band, and traditional music, was limited, though available studies suggested similar risk patterns. The heterogeneity of study designs, participant demographics, and methodological approaches limits the capacity to derive a definitive prevalence estimate of hearing loss among musicians. In the future, research should prioritise well-powered, longitudinal studies incorporating representative samples and standardised audiometric assessments.

Agricultural work environments frequently expose workers to hazardous noise levels from machinery, tools, and livestock operations, placing farmworkers at substantial risk for developing NIHL. Despite this occupational hazard, hearing loss among farmworkers remains an under-studied issue within occupational health research. This oversight is concerning, given the often-limited access farmworkers have to preventive healthcare and audiological services. Coco et al.'s (2025) scoping review addressed this gap by synthesising the available evidence on NIHL in farmworker populations. Specifically, they sought to (1) summarise existing research on the prevalence and characteristics of NIHL in farmworkers; (2) catalogue the instruments and methodologies used to evaluate hearing outcomes; (3) describe testing approaches and their limitations; and (4) provide recommendations for improving future research design and policy in this area.

Coco et al.'s review followed Arksey and O'Malley's scoping review framework and adhered to Preferred Reporting Items for Systematic Reviews and Meta-Analyses (PRISMA) reporting guidelines. Systematic searches were conducted across three databases—PubMed, CINAHL, and Scopus—to retrieve studies examining NIHL in farmworkers. Articles were included if they focused on noise-related hearing loss in this population and employed either objective or subjective measures of hearing function. They identified 57 articles that met their inclusion criteria. Most studies were conducted in North America (n = 32, 56%), particularly within the Midwestern United States of America. Study samples predominantly included white, male farmworkers engaged in crop agriculture. Objective hearing assessments using audiometry were reported in 47 studies (82%), conducted in a range of settings including clinics, hospitals, worksites, and even workers' homes. However, considerable variation in diagnostic criteria for hearing loss across studies hindered cross-study comparability. Among the 14 studies that defined hearing loss as greater than 25 dBs, prevalence rates ranged from 46% to 98%. Additionally, 14 studies used subjective measures of hearing difficulty, often relying on non-standardised, researcher-developed survey items. In these, reported prevalence rates of hearing difficulties reached up to 87%.

Coco et al.'s review confirms that hearing loss is both widespread and persistent among farmworkers, with no evidence of declining prevalence over time. Despite this, methodological inconsistencies and a lack of demographic diversity limit the generalisability of findings. Based on this finding, there is a need for more inclusive research involving diverse farmworker populations and for the development of targeted interventions to mitigate occupational noise exposure. Strengthening hearing conservation strategies in agricultural settings is critical to protecting the long-term auditory health of this vulnerable workforce.

As video gaming becomes an increasingly dominant form of entertainment, concerns have emerged about the potential health risks associated with prolonged and high-volume exposure to digital sound environments. Unlike other leisure activities, gaming often involves sustained and immersive audio experiences, frequently delivered through headphones or high-output speakers. This raises important questions about whether gaming may represent an under-recognised and modifiable risk factor for auditory damage, particularly hearing loss and tinnitus. Despite the biological plausibility of this relationship, research about this topic remains sparse. Dillard et al. (2024) conducted a systematic scoping review to assess the current state of evidence regarding the association between gaming and auditory health outcomes, specifically hearing loss and tinnitus. They performed a comprehensive search during January 2023 across three electronic databases—PubMed, Scopus, and Ovid MEDLINE—for peer-reviewed literature. They also sourced grey literature sources. The timeline of the search spanned from the database's inception until January 2023. Included studies comprised observational research, trials, case studies, or mixed-methods designs published in English, Spanish, or Chinese. To be eligible, studies had to explore the relationship between gaming and outcomes related to hearing loss or tinnitus. A total of 14 peer-reviewed studies met their inclusion criteria, consisting of 11 cohort studies and three non-cohort observational studies. Notably, average sound levels associated with video gaming often approached or surpassed recommended safe exposure thresholds. Participants were reported to engage in gaming for an average of three hours per week. Among the five studies that directly assessed associations between gaming and auditory outcomes, four found statistically significant links between gaming and increased risk of hearing loss or tinnitus. Although the evidence remains limited, current findings suggest that video gaming may constitute a widespread and largely overlooked source of hazardous noise exposure. These findings indicate that many gamers may be at risk for developing permanent hearing damage, including hearing loss and tinnitus.

Hearing loss is a prevalent and multifactorial condition that affects millions of people globally. While age and occupational noise exposure are well-established contributors, emerging research has pointed to a wider range of potential environmental, biological, and lifestyle-related factors. Understanding these associations is crucial for developing comprehensive strategies for prevention, early diagnosis, and intervention. To contribute to this growing field, Xu et al. (2024) systematically synthesised meta-analytic evidence about environmental risk factors, protective factors, and biomarkers associated with hearing loss. Their study also aimed to establish a hierarchy of evidence to determine which associations are most robust and clinically significant. They conducted a systematic search for articles across four major electronic databases—Embase, PubMed, Web of Science, and the Cochrane Library—covering all publications up to 1 June 2023. Studies were included if they provided pooled estimates linking hearing loss to environmental or biological factors.

From an initial pool of 9211 articles, 60 meta-analyses met Xu et al.'s inclusion criteria. These comprised data from over 4.1 million people for environmental and protective factors, and from 173,701 people for biomarker analyses. Their review identified 47 environmental risk or protective factors and 46 potential biomarkers. To assess the strength of evidence, associations were ranked using a tiered classification system. Xu et al.'s umbrella review highlights a range of environmental and physiological contributors to hearing loss, with several factors showing strong or highly suggestive associations. The identification of both modifiable risks—such as noise exposure and smoking—and biological indicators—such as height and immune-related conditions—opens new avenues for public health interventions and clinical research. These findings emphasise the importance of adopting a holistic approach to hearing loss prevention and management that incorporates environmental health, chronic disease control, and early life development.

3.1.2 *Diagnostic Approaches*

Occupational NIHL remains one of the most prevalent and preventable work-related health conditions worldwide. Detecting NIHL in its earliest stages is essential for implementing protective interventions before permanent auditory damage occurs. However, conventional audiometric surveillance, often limited to the 0.5–8 kHz frequency range, may miss the subtle threshold shifts that precede clinically significant hearing loss. Makaruse et al. (2025) critically evaluated the diagnostic sensitivity of various audiometric frequencies and early warning metrics to improve surveillance tools and policies aimed at preventing long-term hearing impairment among noise-exposed workers. Their systematic review aimed to address two key questions in occupational audiology:

1. Which audiometric test frequencies or pure-tone averages are most vulnerable to early threshold shifts from occupational noise exposure, prior to significant hearing damage?
2. Which early warning (flag) metrics are most effective in detecting subtle hearing changes indicative of early-stage NIHL for surveillance purposes?

Systematic searches were conducted in Ovid MEDLINE and Embase from July 2021 to May 2024. From 175 retrieved articles, 18 met their inclusion criteria. Data were analysed to identify hearing threshold levels (HTLs) most susceptible to noise-induced shifts and to assess the sensitivity and specificity of various early detection metrics. Out of the included studies, 10 highlighted the importance of extended high-frequency testing—particularly at 12, 14, and 16 kHz—where HTLs were found to be especially noise-sensitive. Conventional mid-frequency ranges (3–6 kHz) were also recognised as vulnerable to early NIHL. However, commonly used surveillance metrics from agencies such as NIOSH and OSHA demonstrated low diagnostic sensitivity and specificity in their current forms. When modified, these metrics achieved 100% sensitivity and 98% specificity, indicating significant potential for refinement in early detection protocols.

The findings from Makaruse et al.'s study underscore the need for enhanced audiometric surveillance tools, particularly those incorporating extended high-frequency testing, to detect NIHL before irreversible damage occurs. Additionally, existing early flag metrics require adjustment to improve diagnostic performance. Further research is needed to validate optimal frequencies and refine sensitive, evidence-based warning metrics for early occupational hearing loss detection.

Acute sensorineural hearing loss encompasses a range of disorders characterised by the sudden onset of hearing impairment, often requiring urgent diagnosis and management. In response to a growing need for evidence-based clinical protocols, Japan issued its first *"Clinical Practice Guidelines for the Diagnosis and Management of Acute Sensorineural Hearing Loss"*, providing a structured approach to the diagnosis and treatment of these conditions. Kitoh et al.'s (2024) article aimed to enhance the scientific rigour of those guidelines by incorporating a systematic review of recent literature and by outlining evidence-informed therapeutic strategies currently available. Drawing on the findings of the national survey and the systematic literature review, a standardised diagnostic algorithm and a set of recommended treatment pathways were developed. These were articulated in conjunction with specifically formulated clinical questions and corresponding evidence-based recommendations. The revised clinical practice guidelines offer a comprehensive and standardised framework for the diagnosis and management of acute sensorineural hearing loss. It is anticipated that these guidelines will contribute to improved clinical practice and serve as a foundation for future research initiatives in the field of otology and audiological medicine.

A growing body of research has drawn attention to a clinical paradox: individuals who exhibit normal pure-tone audiograms yet report significant difficulty understanding speech in noisy environments. This phenomenon, increasingly recognised as hidden hearing loss (HHL), poses a diagnostic challenge because it eludes detection by conventional audiometric assessments. The underlying pathophysiology is believed to involve cochlear synaptopathy—the degeneration of synapses between inner hair cells and auditory nerve fibres. Shenoy et al. (2025) critically examined emerging diagnostic strategies for HHL that focused on identifying electrophysiological markers of synaptopathy. They conducted a comprehensive literature search across multiple scientific databases to identify studies employing objective electrophysiological techniques to measure auditory synaptopathy. The PRISMA guidelines were followed to establish inclusion criteria and ensure methodological rigour.

They discovered 21 studies that met their inclusion criteria. Diagnostic methodologies encompassed auditory brainstem response (ABR), electrocochleography (EcochG), middle ear muscle reflex (MEMR), and frequency-following response. Findings suggest that indicators of synaptopathy may include attenuated wave I amplitudes in ABR, diminished summating potentials in EcochG, and atypical MEMR responses. Many studies also incorporated behavioural assessments—particularly speech-in-noise tests—alongside electrophysiological measures to enhance diagnostic sensitivity. Among the available techniques, ABR emerged as the most utilised method for evaluating HHL. While ABR, EcochG, and MEMR showed potential as diagnostic tools for cochlear synaptopathy, further comparative research is warranted to establish their relative efficacy. A dual-modality diagnostic approach that integrates behavioural and electrophysiological data may offer the most comprehensive framework for identifying and quantifying hidden hearing loss in clinical populations.

3.2 Conclusion

In summary, the findings from the reviewed studies reveal a persistent underestimation of hearing-related conditions, particularly in underserved or non-traditional populations. While promising diagnostic innovations and public health strategies are emerging, significant gaps remain in standardising methodologies, improving early detection, and implementing equitable hearing conservation programs. Bridging these gaps will require coordinated efforts across disciplines to advance evidence-based policy, foster inclusive research, and reduce the global burden of hearing loss.

References

Coco, L., Fried, M., Loria, O., Vazquez, L., Ekonomo, K., Sanchez, G., Keeney, A. J., & Beseler, C. L. (2025). Noise-induced hearing loss in farmworkers: A scoping review. *Frontiers in Public Health, 13*, 1502489. https://doi.org/10.3389/fpubh.2025.1502489

Dillard, L. K., Mulas, P., Der, C., Fu, X., & Chadha, S. (2024). Risk of sound induced hearing loss from exposure to video gaming or esports: A systematic scoping review. *BMJ Public Health, 2*(1), e000253. https://doi.org/10.1136/bmjph-2023-000253

Firle, C., & Richter, A. H. (2025). A scoping review of the prevalence of musicians' hearing loss. *Frontiers in Public Health, 13*, 1472134. https://doi.org/10.3389/fpubh.2025.1472134

Kitoh, R., Nishio, S. Y., Sato, H., Ikezono, T., Morita, S., Wada, T., Usami, S. I., & Research Group on Intractable Hearing Disorders and Japan Audiological Society. (2024). Clinical practice guidelines for the diagnosis and management of acute sensorineural hearing loss. *Auris, Nasus, Larynx, 51*(4), 811–821. https://doi.org/10.1016/j.anl.2024.06.004

Makaruse, N., Maslin, M. R. D., & Shai Campbell, Z. (2025). Early identification of potential occupational noise-induced hearing loss: A systematic review. *International Journal of Audiology, 64*(5), 419–428. https://doi.org/10.1080/14992027.2024.2418354

Shenoy, S., Bhatt, K., Yazdani, Y., Rahimian, H., Djalilian, H. R., & Abouzari, M. (2025). A systematic review: State of the science on diagnostics of hidden hearing loss. *Diagnostics (Basel, Switzerland), 15*(6), 742. https://doi.org/10.3390/diagnostics15060742

Xu, X., Liao, Y., Zhang, L., He, Y., Zhang, Y., Xiong, D., & Xie, H. (2024). Environmental risk factors, protective factors, and biomarkers for hearing loss: An umbrella review. *Otolaryngology--Head and Neck Surgery: Official Journal of American Academy of Otolaryngology-Head and Neck Surgery, 171*(2), 323–339. https://doi.org/10.1002/ohn.724

Chapter 4
Hearing Loss Across the Lifespan and Cognitive, Psychological, Developmental, and Health Outcomes

4.1 Cognitive, Psychological, and Psychosocial Outcomes Across the Lifespan

4.1.1 Cognitive and Psychological Outcomes

Evidence suggests that hearing loss is not only a sensory deficit but also a factor associated with adverse mental health outcomes and cognitive decline. However, data specific to African populations remain sparse. Ahmed et al. (2025) aimed to address this gap by summarising available research on the associations between hearing loss, mental health, and cognitive function within African contexts.

Ahmed et al.'s systematic review was conducted in accordance with Preferred Reporting Items for Systematic Reviews and Meta-Analyses (PRISMA) guidelines, focusing on cohort, case–control, and cross-sectional studies that compared mental health outcomes or cognitive functioning between people with hearing loss or deafness and those with normal hearing. Their initial search yielded 2822 records from electronic databases. After title, abstract, and full-text screening, seven studies met their eligibility criteria. Most studies involved special populations such as residents of retirement homes and attendees of special schools, with a predominance of female participants. Five studies identified a significant association between hearing loss and increased prevalence of poor mental health outcomes, indicating that hearing impairment may contribute to psychological distress in affected individuals. Their review highlighted an increased risk of mental health disorders and cognitive decline associated with hearing impairment in African populations. Nonetheless, the limited number of studies and their focus on specialised populations suggest a need for further research across more representative groups.

Hearing loss in children is not solely a sensory impairment but a condition that can profoundly affect emotional development, social integration, and psychological

G. Bennett, *Understanding Hearing Loss*, SpringerBriefs in Modern Perspectives on Disability Research,
https://doi.org/10.1007/978-981-95-1096-2_4

health. Previous research has estimated that between 20% and 40% of children with hearing loss experience psychosocial difficulties. However, these figures may no longer accurately reflect current realities, given substantial advances in hearing technologies, early intervention, and rehabilitative care. An updated synthesis of the literature is therefore necessary to assess contemporary risk factors and inform best practices in clinical and educational settings.

de Jong et al. (2024) evaluated and synthesised literature concerning the psychosocial outcomes of children with hearing loss and attempted to identify current predictors that may influence their psychosocial well-being. Their study employed a systematic review methodology. Relevant peer-reviewed articles were identified through comprehensive searches conducted in Embase, Medline, PsycINFO, and the Web of Science Core Collection. Inclusion criteria focused on original research evaluating psychosocial outcomes in children with hearing loss. The methodological quality of included studies was assessed using the Newcastle-Ottawa Quality Assessment Scale and a set of custom reviewers' criteria tailored for this review. They performed a search of the databases on 20 October 2022, which yielded 1561 records. Following screening and eligibility assessment, 36 studies were included for full review. Of these, 24 were rated as of fair to good quality, while 12 were deemed to be of poor methodological quality. de Jong et al. concluded that children with hearing loss were found to have approximately twice the risk of experiencing psychosocial difficulties compared to their peers with typical hearing. Notably, psychosocial outcomes were more accurately predicted by measures of communicative functioning—such as speech perception in noise and language proficiency—than by the degree of hearing impairment itself. These findings underscore the importance of early identification of at-risk children and the implementation of targeted psychological interventions to support their social and emotional development.

Adult-onset hearing loss (AOHL) is increasingly recognised as a modifiable risk factor for dementia. As global populations age, understanding the underlying biological mechanisms linking hearing impairment to neurodegeneration has become a public health imperative. While epidemiological studies have established an association between AOHL and increased dementia risk, the neuropathological pathways remain inadequately understood. Lasica et al.'s (2025) systematic review synthesised current evidence on the relationship between AOHL and biomarkers indicative of Alzheimer's disease and related dementias, including cerebrospinal fluid and blood-based biomarkers, as well as neuroimaging findings. They conducted a systematic search of electronic databases from the database's inception through to 30 April 2024. Eligible studies included cross-sectional and longitudinal analyses reporting quantitative associations between AOHL and biomarkers of dementia. The methodological quality of the studies was appraised using the Mixed Methods Appraisal Tool. Given the heterogeneity in study design and outcome measures, a narrative synthesis was performed.

Lasica et al. identified a total of 66 studies, comprising 63 cross-sectional and 10 longitudinal analyses. Their review reveals that AOHL is frequently associated with grey matter atrophy in temporal brain regions and elevated in vivo tau biomarkers, both cross-sectionally and longitudinally. These findings suggest that neurodegeneration, particularly within medial temporal structures, and tau accumulation may underlie the observed increase in dementia risk among people with AOHL. The results support the hypothesis that AOHL contributes to reduced cognitive reserve, thereby heightening vulnerability to dementia. Future longitudinal, biomarker-focused studies are essential to clarify causality and inform preventative strategies.

Age-related hearing loss (ARHL) is one of the most prevalent chronic conditions affecting older adults globally, and it is increasingly recognised as a factor influencing psychosocial health. Depression is similarly common in later life and contributes significantly to morbidity and reduced quality of life. While epidemiological studies have suggested an association between ARHL and depressive symptoms, the magnitude of this relationship and the moderating roles of demographic variables remain to be clarified. Li et al.'s (2025) meta-analysis synthesises existing evidence to determine the strength of the association between ARHL and depression in older adults, and to examine the potential moderating effects of age and gender. Li et al. performed a systematic literature search within four English-language databases: PubMed, Embase, Web of Science, and the Cochrane Library. They identified nine studies: three longitudinal cohort studies and six cross-sectional studies. Their findings suggest that ARHL is associated with an increased risk of depressive symptoms in older adults, with the relationship being more pronounced among studies with higher female representation. These results underscore the need for integrated audiological and psychological screening in geriatric populations, particularly among older women. Further longitudinal research is warranted to explore causal pathways and inform targeted interventions.

Mild cognitive impairment (MCI), a clinical state that often precedes dementia, represents a critical target for early intervention. Emerging research suggests a correlation between ARHL and elevated risk for MCI, yet the evidence remains heterogeneous. Wu et al.'s (2024) systematic review and meta-analysis aimed to synthesise current findings to clarify the strength and nature of the association between ARHL and the risk of developing MCI, with the goal of informing both clinical practice and preventative strategies. Their review was conducted in accordance with the Preferred Reporting Items for Systematic Reviews and Meta-Analyses (PRISMA) guidelines. Comprehensive searches were undertaken across multiple databases, including the China Knowledge Network, Wanfang, China Biomedical Literature Database, PubMed, Cochrane Library, Embase, and Web of Science. Two reviewers independently performed study selection, quality assessment, and data extraction. In total, 13 studies, encompassing a cumulative total of 2,222,036 individuals, were included in their final analysis. These studies investigated a range of demographic, vascular-neurologic, and psychosocial variables associated with ARHL and cognitive function. Eleven risk factors were identified as significantly associated with an increased likelihood of developing MCI in individuals with ARHL: older age (OR = 1.63; 95% CI: 1.09–2.43), male sex (OR = 1.29; 95% CI: 1.14–1.47), severity of hearing loss (OR = 1.35; 95% CI: 1.03–1.75), non-use of hearing aids (OR = 1.56; 95% CI: 1.37–1.79), cerebrovascular disease (OR = 1.41; 95% CI: 1.17–1.69), cardiovascular disease (OR = 1.29; 95% CI: 1.07–1.55), diabetes mellitus (OR = 1.28; 95% CI: 1.20–1.35), history of head trauma (OR = 1.22; 95% CI: 1.13–1.33), alcohol use (OR = 1.28; 95% CI: 1.14–1.43), tobacco use (OR = 1.19; 95% CI: 1.14–1.25), and presence of depression (OR = 1.63; 95% CI: 1.47–1.81).

Wu et al. concluded that ARHL significantly increases the risk of developing MCI, particularly in the presence of specific demographic, vascular, and psychological comorbidities. These insights support the need for tailored intervention strategies in geriatric care that incorporate hearing assessments and rehabilitative services as part of broader cognitive health monitoring. Early identification and management of these risk factors may contribute to delaying or preventing cognitive decline in the ageing population.

Depression and hearing loss are both common conditions that significantly affect quality of life and public health. While several studies have suggested that hearing loss may increase the risk of developing depression, the consistency and strength of this association have varied across different research contexts. Variability in study designs, follow-up durations, participant age ranges, and cohort methodologies has contributed to uncertainty about the true nature of this relationship. To clarify these inconsistencies, Wei et al. (2024) conducted a meta-analysis of cohort studies examining the link between hearing loss and depression, drawing on a broad base of longitudinal research. An extensive search of the PubMed, Embase, and Cochrane Library databases was undertaken to identify relevant cohort studies. Their final analysis included 24 cohort studies published between 2007 and 2024, encompassing a wide range of sample sizes—from as few as 548 to over 250,000 participants. Across these studies, a total of 24,304 individuals had experienced a depressive episode. The pooled results indicate that hearing loss was associated with a 35% increased risk of depression (OR = 1.35; 95% CI: 1.27–1.44), suggesting a statistically significant and clinically relevant relationship. Taken together, these findings support the conclusion that hearing loss contributes to an elevated risk of depression, independent of other factors. This reinforces the importance of considering hearing loss not just as a sensory issue, but as a broader health concern with implications for mental well-being. Clinicians and public health professionals should be aware of the psychological risks associated with untreated hearing impairment and consider early interventions that address both auditory and emotional health.

The potential association between hearing loss—including both sensorineural impairment and conductive conditions such as otitis media with effusion (OME)—and learning difficulties in children has been a subject of increasing concern within educational and clinical research. Hearing plays a pivotal role in early language acquisition, and delays or deficits in auditory input during critical developmental windows may adversely affect literacy and academic performance. Savegnago et al.'s (2024) synthesised current evidence on the relationship between hearing loss and learning difficulties in paediatric populations and explored associated neuropsychological patterns and risk factors. A comprehensive literature search was conducted using the PubMed, Cochrane, and Scopus databases. Inclusion criteria comprised (i) studies published post-2000, (ii) samples composed of individuals under 18 years of age, (iii) studies that investigated co-occurrence of learning difficulties with hearing loss and/or OME, and (iv) articles published in English.

Exclusion criteria included (i) the presence of comorbid conditions other than hearing loss and/or OME within the study cohort and (ii) non-original research articles. Out of 924 records initially identified, four studies met the inclusion criteria. Key findings include: (i) children with hearing loss who received diagnostic and rehabilitative intervention before 6 months of age demonstrated superior school readiness and enhanced language and literacy skills compared to those who received later intervention; (ii) increased frequency of OME episodes and the presence of conductive hearing loss during the language acquisition phase were associated with reduced reading proficiency; and (iii) reading difficulties observed in children with hearing loss closely resembled those characteristic of broader language impairments. Despite these findings the current evidence base remains limited, highlighting a substantial need for further research exploring the relationship between hearing loss and learning outcomes. In the future, studies should employ robust diagnostic methodologies to identify and characterise reading and writing difficulties among children with varying degrees of hearing loss, across diverse developmental stages.

Hearing loss in adulthood, particularly age-related sensorineural hearing loss, has emerged as a significant modifiable risk factor for cognitive impairment and dementia. While previous meta-analyses have identified an association between hearing loss and adverse cognitive outcomes, they often lacked comprehensiveness regarding dementia subtypes, dose–response relationships, and moderating variables. Yu et al.'s (2024) systematic review and meta-analysis aimed to consolidate cohort-based evidence to evaluate the extent and consistency of these associations and to explore potential moderators and subtype-specific risks. Eligible studies were prospective cohorts with baseline hearing assessments, a minimum follow-up of 2 years, and outcomes of incident cognitive decline or dementia. A total of 50 studies (n = 1,548,754 participants) were included. Their analysis confirmed that adult-onset hearing loss is a robust, independent risk factor for cognitive decline, mild cognitive impairment, and Alzheimer's disease dementia.

4.2 Conclusion

Overall, the evidence confirms that hearing loss is far more than a sensory impairment; it is a significant contributor to mental health challenges, cognitive decline, and developmental delays across different life stages. Key protective factors—such as early diagnosis, timely intervention, and communicative functioning—can mitigate many of these adverse outcomes, underscoring the importance of integrated, person-centred approaches to hearing care. However, current research remains limited in scope and generalisability, particularly in under-represented regions and among diverse populations. Continued longitudinal, interdisciplinary, and biomarker-driven research will be critical to improving clinical practices and shaping effective, evidence-based policies aimed at enhancing quality of life for individuals with hearing loss across the lifespan.

References

Ahmed, A., Tsiga-Ahmed, F., Bello-Muhammad, N., Ajiya, A., Gudaji, M., & Stefler, D. (2025). Association of hearing loss with cognitive function and mental health in Africa: A systematic review. *BMC Public Health, 25*(1), 298. https://doi.org/10.1186/s12889-025-21548-3

de Jong, T. J., van der Schroeff, M. P., Stapersma, L., & Vroegop, J. L. (2024). A systematic review on the impact of auditory functioning and language proficiency on psychosocial difficulties in children and adolescents with hearing loss. *International Journal of Audiology, 63*(9), 675–685. https://doi.org/10.1080/14992027.2023.2261074

Lasica, A. B., Sheppard, J., Yu, R. C., Livingston, G., Ridgway, N., Omar, R., Schilder, A. G. M., & Costafreda, S. G. (2025). Association between adult-onset hearing loss and dementia biomarkers: A systematic review. *Ageing Research Reviews, 104*, 102647. https://doi.org/10.1016/j.arr.2024.102647

Li, F., Jin, M., Ma, T., & Cui, C. (2025). Association between age-related hearing loss and depression: A systematic review and meta-analysis. *PLoS One, 20*(1), e0298495. https://doi.org/10.1371/journal.pone.0298495

Savegnago, D., Franz, L., Gubernale, M., Gallo, C., de Filippis, C., Marioni, G., & Genovese, E. (2024). Learning disabilities in children with hearing loss: A systematic review. *American Journal of Otolaryngology, 45*(5), 104439. https://doi.org/10.1016/j.amjoto.2024.104439

Wei, J., Li, Y., & Gui, X. (2024). Association of hearing loss and risk of depression: A systematic review and meta-analysis. *Frontiers in Neurology, 15*, 1446262. https://doi.org/10.3389/fneur.2024.1446262

Wu, C., Wang, W., Li, R., Su, Y., Lv, H., Qin, S., & Zheng, Z. (2024). Risk factors for mild cognitive impairment in patients with age-related hearing loss: A meta-analysis. *Brazilian Journal of Otorhinolaryngology, 90*(6), 101467. https://doi.org/10.1016/j.bjorl.2024.101467

Yu, R. C., Proctor, D., Soni, J., Pikett, L., Livingston, G., Lewis, G., Schilder, A., Bamiou, D., Mandavia, R., Omar, R., Pavlou, M., Lin, F., Goman, A. M., & Gonzalez, S. C. (2024). Adult-onset hearing loss and incident cognitive impairment and dementia – A systematic review and meta-analysis of cohort studies. *Ageing Research Reviews, 98*, 102346. https://doi.org/10.1016/j.arr.2024.102346

Chapter 5
Opportunities for Research in the Future

5.1 Methodological Limitations in the Studies Reviewed

5.1.1 Language Bias (English-Only Studies)

In the context of the research examined, language bias refers to the systematic exclusion of non-English language studies in literature reviews and meta-analyses. This is a common limitation, as many reviews restrict their inclusion criteria to studies published in English, thereby potentially omitting significant research conducted and published in other languages. This practice skews the evidence base by over-representing findings from English-speaking countries, particularly Western contexts, and under-representing research from non-English-speaking regions that may offer different perspectives or outcomes. As a result, the conclusions drawn from such studies may lack cultural and geographic diversity, limiting their applicability to global populations. To mitigate this limitation, future research should incorporate multilingual search strategies, use translation services where feasible, and collaborate with international scholars to ensure a more inclusive and representative evidence base (see Table 5.1).

5.1.2 Exclusion of Grey Literature and Non-Peer-Reviewed Sources

Many systematic and scoping reviews exclude grey literature—such as government reports, theses, conference proceedings, and technical papers—on the grounds that they have not undergone peer review. While peer-reviewed sources offer a level of quality assurance, excluding grey literature can introduce publication bias, where

G. Bennett, *Understanding Hearing Loss*, SpringerBriefs in Modern Perspectives on Disability Research,
https://doi.org/10.1007/978-981-95-1096-2_5

Table 5.1 Common limitations in the meta-analyses and systematic reviews examined for this book

Limitation identified	References
Language bias (English-only studies)	Ahmed et al. (2025), Coco et al. (2025), de Jong et al. (2024), Frisby et al. (2024), Makaruse et al. (2025), Morvan et al. (2024), Weerapol and Leelakanok (2024)
Exclusion of grey literature and non-peer-reviewed sources	Frisby et al. (2024), Makaruse et al. (2025)
Small sample sizes	Morvan et al. (2024), Wu et al. (2024)
Heterogeneity of methods and measures	Ahmed et al. (2025), de Jong et al. (2024), Dillard et al. (2024), Morvan et al. (2024), Xu et al. (2024)
Lack of standardised outcome measures	de Jong et al. (2024), Morvan et al. (2024)
Lack of meta-analysis or quantitative synthesis	Coco et al. (2025), de Jong et al. (2024), Morvan et al. (2024)
Limited generalisability (e.g. Western or specific institutional samples)	Ahmed et al. (2025), Coco et al. (2025), de Jong et al. (2024), Wu et al. (2024)
No quality assessment in scoping reviews	Coco et al. (2025), Dillard et al. (2024)
Single reviewer bias in screening	Dillard et al. (2024)
Inclusion of observational studies only	Wei et al. (2024), Xu et al. (2024)
Inability to infer causality	Ahmed et al. (2025), Wei et al. (2024), Xu et al. (2024)
Residual confounding	Ahmed et al. (2025), Wei et al.(2024)
Use of self-reported measures	Ahmed et al. (2025)
Lack of regression analyses	Ahmed et al. (2025)
Limited representativeness of hearing loss types	Ahmed et al. (2025), Morvan et al. (2024)
Retrospective study design and recall bias	Wei et al. (2024)

only studies with significant or positive findings are included. This limits the comprehensiveness of the review and potentially overlooks valuable insights, particularly in emerging or under-researched areas. The exclusion of non-peer-reviewed work can also reinforce institutional biases, favouring academic over practitioner or community-based knowledge. Future research can address this limitation by systematically searching grey literature databases and assessing the quality of such sources using adapted appraisal tools to ensure transparency and rigour (see Table 5.1).

5.1.3 Small Sample Sizes

Small sample sizes are a recurring limitation in hearing loss studies, often due to recruitment challenges, resource constraints, or the specific nature of the populations being studied. Studies with small cohorts may lack the statistical power to detect significant effects or generalise findings beyond the sample. This limitation undermines the reliability and external validity of the research and increases the risk of both Type I and Type II errors. Future studies should aim for larger, more diverse samples through multi-site collaborations, use of national databases, or adaptive trial designs that allow for sample size adjustments. Additionally, transparent reporting of power calculations can help readers assess the robustness of the study's conclusions (see Table 5.1).

5.1.4 Heterogeneity of Methods and Measures

The use of varied research designs, measurement tools, and analytical approaches across studies creates a high degree of heterogeneity in hearing loss research. This diversity complicates efforts to compare findings, synthesise data, or draw overarching conclusions. Inconsistencies in how hearing loss is defined, measured, and reported—along with differences in participant demographics and study settings—reduce the coherence of the evidence base. Such heterogeneity hinders meta-analyses and makes it difficult to identify patterns or replicate results. To reduce methodological variability, future research should work towards consensus on standard protocols and core outcome sets while explicitly justifying deviations from established norms (see Table 5.1).

5.1.5 Lack of Standardised Outcome Measures

A significant challenge in the field of hearing research is the lack of standardised outcome measures, which impairs comparability across studies. Researchers often use different tools to assess similar constructs—such as hearing thresholds, quality of life, or communication ability—leading to inconsistent results. This fragmentation limits the feasibility of data synthesis and reduces confidence in the conclusions of individual studies. The absence of standardised outcomes also hinders the accumulation of evidence needed to support policy or clinical guidelines. Mitigation strategies include the development and adoption of validated, universally accepted measurement instruments and the creation of reporting guidelines that mandate the use of core outcomes in hearing loss research (see Table 5.1).

5.1.6 Lack of Meta-Analysis or Quantitative Synthesis

Despite the growing body of literature on hearing loss, many reviews stop short of conducting meta-analyses, often due to heterogeneity or lack of sufficient data. The absence of quantitative synthesis limits the ability to estimate effect sizes, assess heterogeneity statistically, or identify moderating variables. Consequently, readers are left with narrative summaries that may be more prone to subjective interpretation. To address this limitation, future reviews should prioritise meta-analytic techniques wherever possible, even if subgroup analyses or sensitivity checks are needed to account for variability. Where meta-analysis is not feasible, authors should clearly explain why and consider using alternative synthesis methods like meta-regression or vote-counting techniques (see Table 5.1).

5.1.7 Limited Generalisability (e.g. Western or Specific Institutional Samples)

Many studies on hearing loss were conducted in high-income, Western countries or within specific institutional settings, such as university clinics or hospitals. This limited generalisability restricts the applicability of findings to broader, more diverse populations, particularly those in low- and middle-income countries. The homogeneity of samples in terms of geography, socioeconomic status, and cultural background can result in findings that are not reflective of global realities. Future research should seek to diversify study populations by including participants from various geographic regions, ethnicities, and socioeconomic backgrounds. Collaborations with international institutions and community-based participatory research approaches can enhance external validity and relevance (see Table 5.1).

5.1.8 No Quality Assessment in Scoping Reviews

Literature reviews and meta-analyses often omit formal quality appraisal of included studies, since their primary goal is to map the breadth of available evidence rather than to evaluate its validity. However, the lack of quality assessment means that poor-quality studies are given equal weight to high-quality ones, which can distort the synthesis and mislead readers. This is particularly problematic when such studies inform policy or practice. To address this limitation, future studies should incorporate basic quality checks or include an optional appraisal step, clearly distinguishing between the mapping function and critical appraisal to maintain transparency (see Table 5.1).

5.1.9 Single Reviewer Bias in Screening

In some reviews, especially those with limited resources, study screening and data extraction were conducted by a single reviewer. This introduced a risk of bias due to subjective judgement, oversight, or inconsistency in applying inclusion criteria. Single reviewer bias undermines the reliability of the review and may lead to the inclusion or exclusion of inappropriate studies. To mitigate this limitation, reviews should employ at least two independent reviewers at each stage, with a third party available to resolve discrepancies. If only one reviewer is feasible, it is essential to implement detailed protocols, pilot testing, and inter-rater reliability checks to safeguard against single reviewer bias (see Table 5.1).

5.1.10 Inclusion of Observational Studies Only

Many hearing loss reviews are limited to observational studies, which are valuable for exploring associations but are inherently prone to bias and confounding. Without experimental manipulation, these studies cannot definitively establish causality, and their findings may be influenced by uncontrolled variables. This reliance on observational data weakens the evidentiary foundation for clinical and policy decisions. Future research should balance observational findings with experimental designs, such as randomised controlled trials (RCTs), when ethical and practical. When RCTs are not feasible, advanced statistical methods like propensity score matching or instrumental variable analysis can be used to approximate causal inferences (see Table 5.1).

5.1.11 Inability to Infer Causality

Closely related to the reliance on observational studies is the general inability to infer causality from most hearing loss research. Even when strong associations are found, they cannot confirm that one variable causes another without ruling out all possible confounders and reverse causation. This limitation hampers the development of targeted interventions. Future research should prioritise longitudinal designs, quasi-experimental approaches, and triangulation with experimental data to strengthen causal claims. Clear articulation of causal hypotheses and use of frameworks like Bradford Hill criteria can also enhance interpretive rigour (see Table 5.1).

5.1.12 Residual Confounding

Residual confounding occurs when not all relevant variables are measured or adequately controlled for in a study, leaving open the possibility that observed associations are spurious. In hearing loss research, unmeasured factors such as socioeconomic status, environmental exposures, or comorbid conditions may confound results. This limitation undermines the internal validity of the study and can lead to erroneous conclusions. Researchers should attempt to identify and control for as many potential confounders as possible, use robust statistical controls, and consider sensitivity analyses to estimate the impact of unmeasured confounding (see Table 5.1).

5.1.13 Use of Self-Reported Measures

Self-reported data are frequently used in hearing loss research to assess outcomes like hearing ability, psychosocial impact, or service utilisation. While practical and cost-effective, these measures are susceptible to recall bias, social desirability bias, and individual differences in perception. Consequently, they may not accurately reflect objective reality, leading to measurement error. To address this, future research should combine self-reports with objective measures (e.g. audiometry), validate self-report tools against clinical benchmarks, and interpret self-reported data with appropriate caution (see Table 5.1).

5.1.14 Lack of Regression Analyses

In some studies, statistical analyses are limited to descriptive statistics or bivariate comparisons, omitting regression techniques that can adjust for multiple confounding variables. Without regression analyses, it is difficult to isolate the independent effect of key predictors or control for covariates, weakening the explanatory power of the study. Researchers should routinely employ multivariate regression models, clearly report assumptions and diagnostics, and use appropriate modelling techniques based on the data structure (e.g. logistic, linear, or hierarchical models) (see Table 5.1).

5.1.15 Limited Representativeness of Hearing Loss Types

Hearing loss research often fails to account for the heterogeneity of hearing loss types—such as sensorineural, conductive, or mixed—and degrees of severity. Studies that group all types together may obscure important differences in aetiology, experience, and treatment outcomes. This limits the specificity and applicability of research findings. To address this issue, future studies should stratify analyses by type and severity of hearing loss, and clearly define the hearing loss characteristics of their sample. Standardised classification systems should be used to enhance consistency and interpretability (see Table 5.1).

5.1.16 Retrospective Study Design and Recall Bias

Retrospective studies, which rely on participants' recall of past events or data collected for other purposes, are subject to recall bias and missing or inaccurate information. In hearing loss research, this can affect the accuracy of reported onset, treatment history, or exposure to risk factors. Such biases compromise the validity of findings and limit their usefulness for informing future practice. Prospective cohort designs, where data are collected in real time, should be used where possible. When retrospective designs are necessary, triangulating data sources and applying memory aids can help reduce bias (see Table 5.1).

5.2 Conclusion

A nuanced appreciation of the limitations in hearing loss research is essential for interpreting findings responsibly and planning future investigations. The methodological issues outlined in this chapter—ranging from language and selection biases to design-related constraints and analytical omissions—collectively highlight the need for more rigorous, inclusive, and standardised approaches in the field. Addressing these limitations will not only enhance the credibility and generalisability of findings but also support the development of more effective, evidence-based interventions. As the global burden of hearing loss continues to grow, refining our research practices will be crucial to ensuring that the knowledge base truly serves the needs of diverse populations.

References

Ahmed, A., Tsiga-Ahmed, F., Bello-Muhammad, N., Ajiya, A., Gudaji, M., & Stefler, D. (2025). Association of hearing loss with cognitive function and mental health in Africa: A systematic review. *BMC Public Health, 25*(1), 298. https://doi.org/10.1186/s12889-025-21548-3

Coco, L., Fried, M., Loria, O., Vazquez, L., Ekonomo, K., Sanchez, G., Keeney, A. J., & Beseler, C. L. (2025). Noise-induced hearing loss in farmworkers: A scoping review. *Frontiers in Public Health, 13*, 1502489. https://doi.org/10.3389/fpubh.2025.1502489

de Jong, T. J., van der Schroeff, M. P., Stapersma, L., & Vroegop, J. L. (2024). A systematic review on the impact of auditory functioning and language proficiency on psychosocial difficulties in children and adolescents with hearing loss. *International Journal of Audiology, 63*(9), 675–685. https://doi.org/10.1080/14992027.2023.2261074

Dillard, L. K., Mulas, P., Der, C., Fu, X., & Chadha, S. (2024). Risk of sound-induced hearing loss from exposure to video gaming or esports: A systematic scoping review. *BMJ Public Health, 2*(1), e000253. https://doi.org/10.1136/bmjph-2023-000253

Frisby, C., Oosthuizen, I., Manchaiah, V., & Swanepoel, W. (2024). Hearing help-seeking, hearing device uptake and hearing health outcomes in individuals with subclinical hearing loss: A systematic review. *International Journal of Audiology, 63*(12), 925–935. https://doi.org/10.1080/14992027.2024.2311660

Makaruse, N., Maslin, M. R. D., & Shai Campbell, Z. (2025). Early identification of potential occupational noise-induced hearing loss: A systematic review. *International Journal of Audiology, 64*(5), 419–428. https://doi.org/10.1080/14992027.2024.2418354

Morvan, P., Buisson-Savin, J., Boiteux, C., Bailly-Masson, E., Buhl, M., & Thai-Van, H. (2024). Factors in the effective use of hearing aids among subjects with age-related hearing loss: A systematic review. *Journal of Clinical Medicine, 13*(14), 4027. https://doi.org/10.3390/jcm13144027

Weerapol, N., & Leelakanok, N. (2024). Communication between healthcare professionals and patients with hearing loss: A systematic review and meta-analysis. *American Journal of Health-system Pharmacy: AJHP: Official Journal of the American Society of Health-System Pharmacists, 81*(12), 521–530. https://doi.org/10.1093/ajhp/zxae045

Wei, J., Li, Y., & Gui, X. (2024). Association of hearing loss and risk of depression: A systematic review and meta-analysis. *Frontiers in Neurology, 15*, 1446262. https://doi.org/10.3389/fneur.2024.1446262

Wu, C., Wang, W., Li, R., Su, Y., Lv, H., Qin, S., & Zheng, Z. (2024). Risk factors for mild cognitive impairment in patients with age-related hearing loss: A meta-analysis. *Brazilian Journal of Otorhinolaryngology, 90*(6), 101467. https://doi.org/10.1016/j.bjorl.2024.101467

Xu, X., Liao, Y., Zhang, L., He, Y., Zhang, Y., Xiong, D., & Xie, H. (2024). Environmental risk factors, protective factors, and biomarkers for hearing loss: An umbrella review. *Otolaryngology--Head and Neck Surgery: Official Journal of American Academy of Otolaryngology-Head and Neck Surgery, 171*(2), 323–339. https://doi.org/10.1002/ohn.724

Chapter 6
Closing Remarks

Hearing loss is no longer a marginal clinical concern but a far-reaching public health issue with implications across all stages of life. The chapters in this book collectively underscore its complexity—biologically, socially, and culturally—and the pressing need for coordinated, evidence-informed responses. From early developmental delays in children to cognitive decline in older adults, hearing impairment affects individuals' educational, occupational, psychological, and interpersonal outcomes in profound ways.

This book has drawn together a broad spectrum of research to illuminate how current interventions, diagnostic practices, and policy responses are meeting—and at times falling short of—the needs of people with hearing loss. Chapter 2 examined the effectiveness of existing services and technologies, revealing disparities in access and outcomes across life stages and population groups. It highlighted both the strengths and the limitations of current interventions, noting particularly the exclusion of under-researched populations such as individuals with subclinical hearing loss and people with limited English proficiency. These insights call attention to the importance of inclusive, culturally responsive, and tailored approaches to hearing care.

Chapter 3 built on this by examining how environmental, occupational, and sociodemographic contexts influence hearing loss. Diagnostic limitations and under-recognised risk factors were explored, with particular attention to vulnerable groups such as farmworkers and gamers, and to emerging conditions like hidden hearing loss. The diversity of these contexts reveals a fragmented diagnostic landscape that too often fails to capture the full range of auditory experiences and needs, especially in non-traditional or underserved populations.

The psychosocial and developmental consequences of hearing loss were the focus of Chap. 4. It became evident that hearing loss intersects with a range of outcomes—from developmental delays in children to depression and dementia in older adults. These findings reinforce the necessity of early intervention and sustained

G. Bennett, *Understanding Hearing Loss*, SpringerBriefs in Modern Perspectives on Disability Research,
https://doi.org/10.1007/978-981-95-1096-2_6

communicative support as a means of buffering individuals from compounding disadvantages over time. Importantly, the evidence base increasingly suggests that hearing loss must be considered not only as a sensory condition but also as a critical social determinant of health.

Chapter 5 offered a reflective lens on the research landscape itself. Despite the growing volume of studies on hearing loss, the field continues to grapple with recurring methodological challenges. Weak study designs, inconsistent measurement tools, underpowered samples, and a lack of longitudinal data all constrain the reliability and generalisability of findings. These shortcomings limit the translation of evidence into practice and policy, thereby reinforcing gaps in care and understanding. Moving forward, it is imperative that future research prioritise rigour, transparency, and representativeness, particularly for historically excluded populations.

Taken together, the findings in this book support an urgent call for a more integrated, lifespan-oriented approach to hearing care. This approach must be holistic, accounting not only for auditory thresholds and clinical outcomes but also for communication access, social inclusion, and emotional well-being. To achieve this, researchers, clinicians, policy-makers, and communities must work collaboratively to address existing gaps, leverage emerging technologies, and ensure that interventions are grounded in the lived realities of those most affected by hearing loss.

As the global burden of hearing impairment continues to rise, the need for more equitable and effective responses grows ever more critical. This book lays the groundwork for such efforts—not only by mapping current knowledge but by identifying the roadblocks that continue to impede progress. With a clearer understanding of what has been achieved and what remains to be done, we can begin to chart a more inclusive, evidence-informed future for hearing loss research and care.

Appendix A Dataset for the Search Term *"Hearing Impairment"*

PubMed ID	First author	Article title	Citation	Citation included in the study
38788800	Yu RC	Adult-onset hearing loss and incident cognitive impairment and dementia - A systematic review and meta-analysis of cohort studies	*Ageing Res Rev*. 2024 Jul;98:102346. doi: 10.1016/j.arr.2024.102346. Epub 2024 May 23.	Yes
38968877	Kitoh R	Clinical practice guidelines for the diagnosis and management of acute sensorineural hearing loss	*Auris Nasus Larynx*. 2024 Aug;51(4):811-821. doi: 10.1016/j.anl.2024.06.004. Epub 2024 Jul 4.	Yes
38506449	Bhat AM	Prognosis of Bilateral Sudden Sensorineural Hearing Loss: A Systematic Review and Meta-Analysis	*Laryngoscope*. 2024 Sep;134(9):3883-3891. doi: 10.1002/lary.31404. Epub 2024 Mar 20.	
37855096	Romli M	Hearing care services for adults with hearing loss in Malaysia: a scoping review	*Int J Audiol*. 2024 Oct;63(10):753-760. doi: 10.1080/14992027.2023.2270594. Epub 2023 Oct 19.	Yes

G. Bennett, *Understanding Hearing Loss*, SpringerBriefs in Modern Perspectives on Disability Research, https://doi.org/10.1007/978-981-95-1096-2

PubMed ID	First author	Article title	Citation	Citation included in the study
38970134	Patil V	A systematic review on the contribution of DNA methylation to hearing loss	*Clin Epigenetics.* 2024 Jul 5;16(1):88. doi: 10.1186/s13148-024-01697-9.	
39068816	Savegnago D	Learning disabilities in children with hearing loss: A systematic review	*Am J Otolaryngol.* 2024 Sep-Oct;45(5):104439. doi: 10.1016/j.amjoto.2024.104439. Epub 2024 Jul 24.	Yes
38956759	Mills JF	Charcot-Marie-Tooth Disease and Hearing Loss: A Systematic Review With Meta-Analysis	*Otol Neurotol.* 2024 Aug 1;45(7):732-739. doi: 10.1097/MAO.0000000000004243. Epub 2024 Jul 2.	
39193144	Liu X	Efficacy of hyperbaric oxygen therapy in treating sudden sensorineural hearing loss: an umbrella review	*Front Neurol.* 2024 Aug 13;15:1453055. doi: 10.3389/fneur.2024.1453055. eCollection 2024.	
39012479	Alper L	Idiopathic sudden sensorineural hearing loss after COVID-19 vaccination: a systematic review and meta-analysis	*Eur Arch Otorhinolaryngol.* 2024 Dec;281(12):6275-6281. doi: 10.1007/s00405-024-08839-y. Epub 2024 Jul 16.	
38895947	Hao Y	Diagnosis and Management of Unexplained Conductive Hearing Loss With Intact Tympanic Membrane: A Systematic Review	*Ear Nose Throat J.* 2024 Jun 19:1455613241262129. doi: 10.1177/01455613241262129. Online ahead of print.	

(continued)

PubMed ID	First author	Article title	Citation	Citation included in the study
38808803	Ying YM	Natural History of Untreated Idiopathic Sudden Sensorineural Hearing Loss	*Laryngoscope*. 2024 Sep;134 Suppl 9:S1-S15. doi: 10.1002/lary.31474. Epub 2024 May 29.	
38411671	Corazzi V	Late-onset, progressive sensorineural hearing loss in the paediatric population: a systematic review	*Eur Arch Otorhinolaryngol*. 2024 Jul;281(7):3397-3421. doi: 10.1007/s00405-024-08527-x. Epub 2024 Feb 27.	
39356749	Gu L	The association between thyroid disease and hearing loss: a meta-analysis	*Acta Otolaryngol*. 2024 Sep;144(9):495-502. doi: 10.1080/00016489.2024.2404614. Epub 2024 Oct 2.	
39263638	Hindhede AL	Disparities between objectively measured hearing loss and subjectively perceived aided hearing loss: A scoping review	*SAGE Open Med*. 2024 Sep 9;12:20503121241279230. doi: 10.1177/20503121241279230. eCollection 2024.	
39312737	Ramesh sankar S	Ototoxic Drug Exposure and Hearing Loss in Neonates: A Scoping Review	*Am J Audiol*. 2024 Dec 2;33(4):1356-1377. doi: 10.1044/2024_AJA-24-00065. Epub 2024 Sep 23.	
39274256	Manuelli M	Unilateral Hearing Loss and Auditory Asymmetry in Mitochondrial Disease: A Scoping Review	*J Clin Med*. 2024 Aug 26;13(17):5044. doi: 10.3390/jcm13175044.	
39792720	Diaz-Ordoñez L	Hearing loss in patients with Morquio A syndrome: A scoping review	*Medicine (Baltimore)*. 2025 Jan 10;104(2):e41128. doi: 10.1097/MD.0000000000041128.	

(continued)

PubMed ID	First author	Article title	Citation	Citation included in the study
39064066	Morvan P	Factors in the Effective Use of Hearing Aids among Subjects with Age-Related Hearing Loss: A Systematic Review	*J Clin Med.* 2024 Jul 10;13(14):4027. doi: 10.3390/jcm13144027.	Yes
40098797	Coco L	Noise-induced hearing loss in farmworkers: a scoping review	*Front Public Health.* 2025 Mar 3;13:1502489. doi: 10.3389/fpubh.2025.1502489. eCollection 2025.	Yes
39497727	Wei J	Association of hearing loss and risk of depression: a systematic review and meta-analysis	*Front Neurol.* 2024 Oct 21;15:1446262. doi: 10.3389/fneur.2024.1446262. eCollection 2024.	Yes
38375662	Frisby C	Hearing help-seeking, hearing device uptake and hearing health outcomes in individuals with subclinical hearing loss: a systematic review	*Int J Audiol.* 2024 Dec;63(12):925-935. doi: 10.1080/14992027.2024.2311660. Epub 2024 Feb 20.	Yes
38270208	Yélamos Lorente MÁ	A Systematic Review on Heritability of Sudden Sensorineural Hearing Loss	*Laryngoscope.* 2024 Aug;134(8):3447-3457. doi: 10.1002/lary.31308. Epub 2024 Jan 25.	
39965236	Briggs EE	Preventing Cisplatin-Induced Hearing Loss in Adults: A Systematic Review and Meta-Analysis	*Otol Neurotol.* 2025 Apr 1;46(4):351-357. doi: 10.1097/MAO.0000000000004446. Epub 2025 Feb 4.	
39079457	Wu C	Risk factors for mild cognitive impairment in patients with age-related hearing loss: a meta-analysis	*Braz J Otorhinolaryngol.* 2024 Nov-Dec;90(6):101467. doi: 10.1016/j.bjorl.2024.101467. Epub 2024 Jul 11.	Yes

(continued)

PubMed ID	First author	Article title	Citation	Citation included in the study
39937593	Emamzadehashemi KR	Prevalence of Hearing Loss After Open-Heart Surgery: A Systematic Review	*Braz J Cardiovasc Surg*. 2025 Feb 12;40(1):e20230197. doi: 10.21470/1678-9741-2023-0197.	
39334764	Santaolalla Sanchez FJ	Pathogenesis and New Pharmacological Approaches to Noise-Induced Hearing Loss: A Systematic Review	*Antioxidants (Basel)*. 2024 Sep 12;13(9):1105. doi: 10.3390/antiox13091105.	
40165641	Kallenberger EM	Preventing Hearing Loss in Children Receiving Cisplatin: A Systematic Review and Meta-Analysis	*Laryngoscope*. 2025 Apr 1. doi: 10.1002/lary.32158. Online ahead of print.	
38520228	Xu X	Environmental Risk Factors, Protective Factors, and Biomarkers for Hearing Loss: An Umbrella Review	*Otolaryngol Head Neck Surg*. 2024 Aug;171(2):323-339. doi: 10.1002/ohn.724. Epub 2024 Mar 23.	Yes
38985787	Mittal R	Diabetes mellitus, hearing loss, and therapeutic interventions: A systematic review of insights from preclinical animal models	*PLoS One*. 2024 Jul 10;19(7):e0305617. doi: 10.1371/journal.pone.0305617. eCollection 2024.	
40017553	Firle C	A scoping review of the prevalence of musicians' hearing loss	*Front Public Health*. 2025 Feb 13;13:1472134. doi: 10.3389/fpubh.2025.1472134. eCollection 2025.	Yes
39936645	Migliorelli A	Hearing Loss and Turner Syndrome: A Scoping Review	*J Int Adv Otol*. 2025 Jan 27;21(1):1-6. doi: 10.5152/iao.2025.241723.	

(continued)

PubMed ID	First author	Article title	Citation	Citation included in the study
38430534	Weerapol N	Communication between healthcare professionals and patients with hearing loss: A systematic review and meta-analysis	*Am J Health Syst Pharm.* 2024 Jun 11;81(12):521-530. doi: 10.1093/ajhp/zxae045.	Yes
39707599	Tao Y	The Prevalence and Related Factors of Hearing Loss Among Adults: A Systematic Review and Meta-Analyses	*Ann Otol Rhinol Laryngol.* 2025 Feb;134(2):93-101. doi: 10.1177/00034894241293045. Epub 2024 Oct 22.	
39765013	Aljabri SF	Consanguinity and hearing loss prevalence among Saudi Arabia population	*Int J Pediatr Otorhinolaryngol.* 2025 Feb;189:112209. doi: 10.1016/j.ijporl.2024.112209. Epub 2024 Dec 24.	
40103444	Zhang Z	How to Break Stubborn Association Between Hearing Loss and Cognitive Impairment: A Systematic Review and Meta-Analysis of Moderators and Mediators	*J Geriatr Psychiatry Neurol.* 2025 Mar 19:8919887251328880. doi: 10.1177/08919887251328880. Online ahead of print.	
39839866	Jin X	Association between hypertension and hearing loss: a systemic review and meta-analysis	*Front Neurol.* 2025 Jan 7;15:1470997. doi: 10.3389/fneur.2024.1470997. eCollection 2024.	
39299718	Paing A	Natural history of otitis media with effusion-related hearing loss in children under 12 years: a systematic review	*Arch Dis Child.* 2024 Dec 13;110(1):38-44. doi: 10.1136/archdischild-2024-327463.	

(continued)

PubMed ID	First author	Article title	Citation	Citation included in the study
40111358	Yeo BSY	Hearing Loss and Falls: A Systematic Review and Meta-Analysis	*JAMA Otolaryngol Head Neck Surg*. 2025 May 1;151(5):485-494. doi: 10.1001/jamaoto.2025.0056.	
39856661	Ahmed A	Association of hearing loss with cognitive function and mental health in Africa: A systematic review	*BMC Public Health*. 2025 Jan 24;25(1):298. doi: 10.1186/s12889-025-21548-3.	Yes
40323123	Li J	Physical Activity, Physical Fitness for Hearing Loss in Adults: A Systematic Review	*Laryngoscope*. 2025 May 5. doi: 10.1002/lary.32237. Online ahead of print.	
38251843	Lin CY	Salvage therapy for refractory sudden sensorineural hearing loss (RSSNHL): a systematic review and network meta-analysis	*Int J Audiol*. 2025 Jan;64(1):1-10. doi: 10.1080/14992027.2024.2303037. Epub 2024 Jan 22.	
38787321	Patro C	The Not-So-Slight Perceptual Consequences of Slight Hearing Loss in School-Age Children: A Scoping Review	*Lang Speech Hear Serv Sch*. 2024 Jul;55(3):1002-1022. doi: 10.1044/2024_LSHSS-23-00165. Epub 2024 May 24.	
38836828	Silva BCS	The effects of auditory stimulation on heart rate variability in healthy individuals with normal hearing and with hearing loss: a systematic review and meta-analysis	*Codas*. 2024 May 31;36(4):e20230111. doi: 10.1590/2317-1782/20242023111en. eCollection 2024.	

(continued)

PubMed ID	First author	Article title	Citation	Citation included in the study
39367221	Fernández-Rueda M	Risk factors associated with late-onset hearing loss in children with congenital cytomegalovirus: a systematic review	*Eur Arch Otorhinolaryngol.* 2025 Apr;282(4):1659-1676. doi: 10.1007/s00405-024-09013-0. Epub 2024 Oct 4.	
40176752	Skare TL	Hearing Loss in Connective Tissue Diseases: A Systematic Review	*Eur J Rheumatol.* 2025 Mar 10;12(1):1-24. doi: 10.5152/eurjrheum.2025.23076.	
37887640	de Jong TJ	A systematic review on the impact of auditory functioning and language proficiency on psychosocial difficulties in children and adolescents with hearing loss	*Int J Audiol.* 2024 Sep;63(9):675-685. doi: 10.1080/14992027.2023.2261074. Epub 2023 Oct 27.	Yes
39797597	Rodrigues J	Exploring the Intricate Connection Between Vitamin B12 Deficiency and Hearing Loss: A Systematic Literature Review	*Ear Nose Throat J.* 2025 Jan 11:1455613241298070. doi: 10.1177/01455613241298070. Online ahead of print.	
39092923	Muñoz K	A systematic review of the prevalence of late identified hearing loss in childhood	*Int J Audiol.* 2025 Feb;64(2):103-110. doi: 10.1080/14992027.2024.2385550. Epub 2024 Aug 2.	

(continued)

PubMed ID	First author	Article title	Citation	Citation included in the study
40346847	Théorêt K	Systematic Review of Quality of Life in Bone Anchored Hearing: Conductive vs. Unilateral Sensorineural Hearing Loss	*Laryngoscope*. 2025 May 10. doi: 10.1002/lary.32229. Online ahead of print.	
40150638	Wang J	Association Between In-Utero Exposure to Antibiotics and Offspring's Hearing Loss: A Systematic Review and Meta-Analysis	*Children (Basel)*. 2025 Mar 13;12(3):356. doi: 10.3390/children12030356.	
40343450	Khadivi A	Proton pump inhibitors and risk of hearing loss; a systematic review	*Naunyn Schmiedebergs Arch Pharmacol*. 2025 May 9. doi: 10.1007/s00210-025-04241-5. Online ahead of print.	
39931625	Henao Rincón MA	Exploring the Potential of Stem Cells: A Systematic Review on Cellular Therapy for Sensorineural Hearing Loss	*Cureus*. 2025 Jan 11;17(1):e77286. doi: 10.7759/cureus.77286. eCollection 2025 Jan.	
39746404	Lasica AB	Association between adult-onset hearing loss and dementia biomarkers: A systematic review	*Ageing Res Rev*. 2025 Feb;104:102647. doi: 10.1016/j.arr.2024.102647. Epub 2024 Dec 31.	Yes
40108599	Mbhele S	Clinical balance assessment tools for children with hearing loss: a scoping review	*BMC Pediatr*. 2025 Mar 19;25(1):218. doi: 10.1186/s12887-025-05563-2.	

(continued)

PubMed ID	First author	Article title	Citation	Citation included in the study
40094897	Di Stadio A	"Do You Hear What I Hear?" Speech and Voice Alterations in Hearing Loss: A Systematic Review	*J Clin Med*. 2025 Feb 20;14(5):1428. doi: 10.3390/jcm14051428.	
38956802	Thompson-Harvey A	Effect of Non-ablative Medical Therapy on Progression of Hearing Loss in Menière's Disease: A Systematic Review and meta-Analysis	*Otol Neurotol*. 2024 Sep 1;45(8):833-839. doi: 10.1097/MAO.0000000000004251. Epub 2024 Jul 3.	
39252156	González-García M	Auditory Prognosis of Patients With Sudden Sensorineural Hearing Loss in Relation to the Presence of Acute Vestibular Syndrome: A Systematic Literature Review and Meta-Analysis	*Ear Hear*. 2025 Jan-Feb 01;46(1):8-15. doi: 10.1097/AUD.0000000000001576. Epub 2024 Sep 10.	
39752630	Li F	Association between age-related hearing loss and depression: A systematic review and meta-analysis	*PLoS One*. 2025 Jan 3;20(1):e0298495. doi: 10.1371/journal.pone.0298495. eCollection 2025.	Yes
39468424	Makaruse N	Early identification of potential occupational noise-induced hearing loss: a systematic review	*Int J Audiol*. 2025 May;64(5):419-428. doi: 10.1080/14992027.2024.2418354. Epub 2024 Oct 28.	Yes

(continued)

PubMed ID	First author	Article title	Citation	Citation included in the study
39679433	Ren W	The efficacy and safety of acupuncture in the treatment of sudden sensorineural hearing loss: A systematic review and meta-analysis	*Integr Med Res*. 2024 Dec;13(4):101087. doi: 10.1016/j.imr.2024.101087. Epub 2024 Sep 21.	
37855793	Murphy B	Modeling the Risk of Hearing Loss From Radiation Therapy in Childhood Cancer Survivors: A PENTEC Comprehensive Review	*Int J Radiat Oncol Biol Phys*. 2024 Jun 1;119(2):446-456. doi: 10.1016/j.ijrobp.2023.08.016. Epub 2023 Oct 19.	
40258119	Arráez Vera G	The Effectiveness of Linguistic Intervention in Children With Hearing Loss: A Systematic Review and Meta-Analysis	*J Speech Lang Hear Res*. 2025 May 8;68(5):2656-2673. doi: 10.1044/2025_JSLHR-24-00589. Epub 2025 Apr 21.	Yes
39543830	Chowdhury A	Older Aboriginal and Torres Strait Islander People's Experiences With Hearing Loss and Audiological Services: A Scoping Review	*Clin Otolaryngol*. 2025 Mar;50(2):191-204. doi: 10.1111/coa.14254. Epub 2024 Nov 14.	
40018090	Dillard LK	Risk of sound-induced hearing loss from exposure to video gaming or esports: a systematic scoping review	*BMJ Public Health*. 2024 Jan 4;2(1):e000253. doi: 10.1136/bmjph-2023-000253. eCollection 2024 Jun.	Yes

(continued)

PubMed ID	First author	Article title	Citation	Citation included in the study
38861427	Bharadwaj SV	Consideration of Demographic Variables in Behavioral Interventions Pertaining to Children With Hearing Loss: A Systematic Review	*Am J Audiol.* 2024 Sep 3;33(3):991-1007. doi: 10.1044/2024_AJA-23-00208. Epub 2024 Jun 11.	
39627856	Berezovsky AN	Cardiovascular Diseases and Sensorineural Hearing Loss-A Systematic Review of the Literature	*Otol Neurotol.* 2025 Jan 1;46(1):23-30. doi: 10.1097/ MAO.0000000000004380. Epub 2024 Nov 21.	
38896785	Tena-García B	Economic Analysis of Cochlear Implants in Adults With Bilateral Severe-to-Profound Hearing Loss. A Systematic Review of the Literature	*Otol Neurotol.* 2024 Aug 1;45(7):717-731. doi: 10.1097/ MAO.0000000000004225. Epub 2024 Jun 18.	
40323204	Plane J	N-acetylcysteine for the Prevention of Cisplatin-Induced Hearing Loss: A Systematic Review and Meta-analysis	*Otolaryngol Head Neck Surg.* 2025 May 5. doi: 10.1002/ohn.1272. Online ahead of print.	
40226262	Balunathan N	Gene-Polymorphism in Non - Syndromic Hearing Loss: A Systematic Review	*Indian J Otolaryngol Head Neck Surg.* 2025 Apr;77(4):1981-1986. doi: 10.1007/s12070-025-05391-x. Epub 2025 Feb 27.	
40150084	Shenoy S	A Systematic Review: State of the Science on Diagnostics of Hidden Hearing Loss	*Diagnostics (Basel).* 2025 Mar 16;15(6):742. doi: 10.3390/ diagnostics15060742.	Yes

(continued)

PubMed ID	First author	Article title	Citation	Citation included in the study
39902389	Di X	Influential publications in sudden hearing loss: a bibliometric and visual synopsis of the top 100 cited articles	*Front Neurol.* 2025 Jan 20;15:1494936. doi: 10.3389/fneur.2024.1494936. eCollection 2024.	
39720938	Chen TY	Association of Polycystic Ovary Syndrome With Sensorineural Hearing Loss: A Systematic Review and Meta-analysis	*Otolaryngol Head Neck Surg.* 2025 Apr;172(4):1121-1132. doi: 10.1002/ohn.1081. Epub 2024 Dec 25.	
39118242	Ferraro T	Use of Speech-to-Text Translation Resources to Address Communication Barriers in Patients With Hearing Loss: A Systematic Review	*Otol Neurotol.* 2024 Oct 1;45(9):961-970. doi: 10.1097/MAO.0000000000004272. Epub 2024 Aug 5.	Yes
39566190	Sohmer J	Health disparities and health literacy challenges experienced by individuals with hearing loss: A scoping review	*Patient Educ Couns.* 2025 Feb;131:108549. doi: 10.1016/j.pec.2024.108549. Epub 2024 Nov 17.	
39863423	Moreno-Herraiz N	Efficacy of Apheresis in the Remission of Sudden Sensorineural Hearing Loss: A Systematic Review and Meta-Analysis	*Clin Ther.* 2025 Apr;47(4):307-315. doi: 10.1016/j.clinthera.2024.12.016. Epub 2025 Jan 24.	

(continued)

PubMed ID	First author	Article title	Citation	Citation included in the study
39074081	Lim TZ	Instruments for evaluating the parental emotional status and ecological support systems among parents who considered cochlear implantation for their children with hearing loss: A scoping review	*PLoS One*. 2024 Jul 29;19(7):e0305748. doi: 10.1371/journal.pone.0305748. eCollection 2024.	
39433333	Paing A	Natural history of otitis media with effusion without hearing loss in children under 12 years: a systematic review	*Arch Dis Child*. 2025 Feb 19;110(3):197-202. doi: 10.1136/archdischild-2024-327464.	
39285307	Patil V	Correction: A systematic review on the contribution of DNA methylation to hearing loss	*Clin Epigenetics*. 2024 Sep 16;16(1):129. doi: 10.1186/s13148-024-01733-8.	
39970981	Han B	Global prevalence of the mitochondrial MT-RNR1 A1555G variant in non-syndromic hearing loss: A systematic review and meta analysis	*Neuroscience*. 2025 Mar 27;570:16-26. doi: 10.1016/j.neuroscience.2025.02.036. Epub 2025 Feb 17.	
38713815		Correction to: Communication between healthcare professionals and patients with hearing loss: A systematic review and meta-analysis	*Am J Health Syst Pharm*. 2024 Jun 24;81(13):e335. doi: 10.1093/ajhp/zxae117.	

(continued)

PubMed ID	First author	Article title	Citation	Citation included in the study
38858237	Fusetti C	Neurobrucellosis Presenting with Motor Damage or Hearing Loss, and Use of Steroids are Associated with a Higher Risk of Sequelae or Relapse: A Systematic Review of Individual Participant Data	*Neurol Sci*. 2024 Nov;45(11):5441-5448. doi: 10.1007/s10072-024-07621-6. Epub 2024 Jun 11.	
40373691	Piva de Freitas P	Quality of life in children with unilateral hearing loss undergoing cochlear implantation: A systematic review and meta-analysis	*Braz J Otorhinolaryngol*. 2025 May 14;91(5):101628. doi: 10.1016/j.bjorl.2025.101628. Online ahead of print.	
40181675	Fouweather M	A systematic review of SARS-CoV-2 associated sudden onset sensorineural hearing loss	*J Laryngol Otol*. 2025 Apr 4:1-15. doi: 10.1017/S002221512500026X. Online ahead of print.	
40021134	Jiang W	Effects of Auditory Training on Cognition in Hearing Loss: A Systematic Review and Meta-analyses	*J Am Acad Audiol*. 2025 Feb 28. doi: 10.3766/jaaa.240049. Online ahead of print.	
40202038	Vagevuur JJ	[Occupational noise-induced hearing loss among dental personnel a scoping review]	*Ned Tijdschr Tandheelkd*. 2025 Apr 7;132(4):180-185. doi: 10.5177/ntvt.2025.04.24097.	

(continued)

PubMed ID	First author	Article title	Citation	Citation included in the study
40059758	Thompson-Harvey A	Reply to the Commentary on "Effect of Non-ablative Medical Therapy on Progression of Hearing Loss in Menière's Disease: A Systematic Review and Meta-Analysis"	*Otol Neurotol.* 2025 Feb 19. doi: 10.1097/MAO.0000000000004465. Online ahead of print.	

Notes:
Search conducted on 19 May 2025
Search terms: (*"hearing impairment"* [Title])
Date range of citations: 1 January 2020 to 19 May 2025
Language of citations: English

Index

G. Bennett, *Understanding Hearing Loss*, SpringerBriefs in Modern Perspectives on Disability Research, https://doi.org/10.1007/978-981-95-1096-2

MIX
Papier aus verantwortungsvollen Quellen
Paper from responsible sources
FSC® C105338

If you have any concerns about our products,
you can contact us on
ProductSafety@springernature.com

In case Publisher is established outside the EU,
the EU authorized representative is:
Springer Nature Customer Service Center GmbH
Europaplatz 3, 69115 Heidelberg, Germany

Printed by Libri Plureos GmbH
in Hamburg, Germany